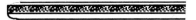

Bruce A. Berger, Ph
Editor

MW01098972

Promoting Civility
in Pharmacy Education

Promoting Civility in Pharmacy Education has been co-published simultaneously as *Journal of Pharmacy Teaching*, Volume 9, Number 3 2002.

Pre-publication
REVIEWS,
COMMENTARIES,
EVALUATIONS . . .

"A MUST-READ for all who teach and supervise pharmacy students. Whether teaching to large classes, small groups, experiential learning, or graduate students, this book offers insight into integrating proper student behavior, pre-professional expectations, and student/faculty interactions. . . . The chapters on promoting civility from the perspective of the new faculty member and on boundary violations in student/faculty relationships are especially valuable, as are the case studies and scenarios depicting common problems that may result in uncivil interactions and possible solutions."

Gerald E. Schumacher, Pharm.D., Ph.D.
Professor of Pharmacy
Northeastern University

More pre-publication
REVIEWS, COMMENTARIES, EVALUATIONS . . .

"WILL APPEAL TO FACULTY interested in creating learning environments that encourage
not only polite behavior but patient-
oriented professional roles and responsibilities. . . . Explores causes of
and cures for incivility in this new
academic environment. Though the
authors do provide strategies for increasing civility in large classrooms,
small groups, experiential programs,
and graduate education, the book's
eight essays are not merely lists of
schoolmarm-ish techniques for crowd
control. They explore deeper moral
issues, demonstrating that the pro-
motion of educational civility involves
the practice, modeling, and inculca-
tion of professional responsibilities."

Thomas D. Zlatic, Ph.D.
Professor of English
Director of the Norton Writing Center
St. Louis College of Pharmacy

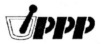

Pharmaceutical Products Press
An Imprint of The Haworth Press, Inc.

Promoting Civility in Pharmacy Education

Promoting Civility in Pharmacy Education has been co-published simultaneously as *Journal of Pharmacy Teaching*, Volume 9, Number 3 2002.

The *Journal of Pharmacy Teaching* Monographic "Separates"

Below is a list of "separates," which in serials librarianship means a special issue simultaneously published as a special journal issue or double-issue *and* as a "separate" hardbound monograph. (This is a format which we also call a "DocuSerial.")

"Separates" are published because specialized libraries or professionals may wish to purchase a specific thematic issue by itself in a format which can be separately cataloged and shelved, as opposed to purchasing the journal on an on-going basis. Faculty members may also more easily consider a "separate" for classroom adoption.

"Separates" are carefully classified separately with the major book jobbers so that the journal tie-in can be noted on new book order slips to avoid duplicate purchasing.

You may wish to visit Haworth's website at . . .

http://www.HaworthPress.com

. . . to search our online catalog for complete tables of contents of these separates and related publications.

You may also call 1-800-HAWORTH (outside US/Canada: 607-722-5857), or Fax 1-800-895-0582 (outside US/Canada: 607-771-0012), or e-mail at:

docdelivery@haworthpress.com

Promoting Civility in Pharmacy Education, edited by Bruce A. Berger, Ph.D., R.Ph. (Vol. 9, No. 3, 2002). *"A MUST-READ for all who teach and supervise pharmacy students." (Gerald E. Schumacher, Pharm.D., Ph.D., Professor of Pharmacy, Northeastern University)*

Handbook for Pharmacy Educators: Getting Adjusted As a New Pharmacy Faculty Member, edited by Shane P. Desselle, Ph.D., and Dana P. Hammer, Ph.D. (Vol. 9, No. 1, 2002). *Helps new pharmacy faculty make a smooth transition into academia.*

Handbook for Pharmacy Educators: Contemporary Teaching Principles and Strategies, edited by Noel E. Wilkin, R.Ph., Ph.D. (Vol. 7, No. 3/4, 2000). *The Handbook for Pharmacy Educators will help you develop ways to delineate and assess outcomes projected by the curricula in order to become an effective teacher amidst the changing health care environment. Also for graduate students, this guide offers an abilities-based approach, provides contemporary strategies for facilitating ability acquisition, and describes the process of assessment that will provide feedback regarding the effectiveness of these teaching strategies. Comprehensive and thorough, this book will help you understand the principles of outcome identification and implementation; strategies that will assist you in teaching students the knowledge, skills, and attitudes associated with those outcomes; the principles of assessment-as- learning; and the process of institutionalization of assessment. The Handbook for Pharmacy Educators will help you implement new teaching methods or rethink old ones to successfully face questions and challenges in the dynamic field of pharmacy.*

Teaching and Learning Strategies in Pharmacy Ethics, Second Edition, edited by Amy Marie Haddad, Ph.D. (Vol. 6, No. 1/2, 1997). *"Offers widened access to creative, invigorating scholarship. . . . It is a window into how instruction in the theory and practice of ethical pharmacy practice meets disparate needs in the contemporary academy." (Jonathan J. Wolfe, PhD, Associate Professor of Pharmacy Practice, University of Arkansas for Medical Sciences, Little Rock)*

Ethical Dimensions of Pharmaceutical Care, edited by Amy Marie Haddad, Ph.D., and Robert A. Buerki, Ph.D. (Vol. 5, No. 1/2, 1996). *"Offers a philosophical basis for understanding just what 'care' is, why the profession ought to care about its patients, and different ways of viewing ethical standards in evaluating pharmaceutical care situations. . . . Balances hard, thought-provoking material with situations requiring applied ethics. . . . Aimed at the foundation of pharmacy's future." (American Journal of Pharmaceutical Education)*

Multicultural Pharmaceutical Education, edited by Barry Bleidt, Ph.D. (Vol. 3, No. 2, 1992). *"Provides practical information on programs that have worked in colleges of pharmacy. Useful reading for those who would like to see their pharmacy schools place greater emphasis on multicultural education and for those who question such efforts." (The Annals of Pharmacotherapy)*

Promoting Civility in Pharmacy Education

Bruce A. Berger, Ph.D., R.Ph.
Editor

Promoting Civility in Pharmacy Education has been co-published simultaneously as *Journal of Pharmacy Teaching*, Volume 9, Number 3 2002.

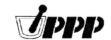

Pharmaceutical Products Press
An Imprint of
The Haworth Press, Inc.
New York • London • Oxford

Published by

Pharmaceutical Products Press®, 10 Alice Street, Binghamton, NY 13904-1580 USA

Pharmaceutical Products Press® is an imprint of The Haworth Press, Inc., 10 Alice Street, Binghamton, NY 13904-1580 USA.

Promoting Civility in Pharmacy Education has been co-published simultaneously as *Journal of Pharmacy Teaching*, Volume 9, Number 3 2002.

© 2003 by The Haworth Press, Inc. All rights reserved. No part of this work may be reproduced or utilized in any form or by any means, electronic or mechanical, including photocopying, microfilm and recording, or by any information storage and retrieval system, without permission in writing from the publisher. Printed in the United States of America.

The development, preparation, and publication of this work has been undertaken with great care. However, the publisher, employees, editors, and agents of The Haworth Press and all imprints of The Haworth Press, Inc., including The Haworth Medical Press® and Pharmaceutical Products Press®, are not responsible for any errors contained herein or for consequences that may ensue from use of materials or information contained in this work. Opinions expressed by the author(s) are not necessarily those of The Haworth Press, Inc. With regard to case studies, identities and circumstances of individuals discussed herein have been changed to protect confidentiality. Any resemblance to actual persons, living or dead, is entirely coincidental.

Cover design by Marylouise E. Doyle

Library of Congress Cataloging-in-Publication Data

Promoting civility in pharmacy education / Bruce A. Berger, editor.
     p. cm.
    "Co-published simultaneously as Journal of pharmacy teaching, vol. 9, no. 3, 2002."
    Includes bibliographical references and index.
    ISBN 0-7890-2120-X (hbk. : alk. paper) – ISBN 0-7890-2121-8 (soft : alk. paper)
    1. Pharmacy–Study and teaching. 2. Courtesy. I. Berger, Bruce A. II. Journal of pharmacy teaching.
RS101 .P76 2003
615'.1'0711–dc21

                       2003005557

Indexing, Abstracting & Website/Internet Coverage

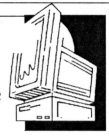

This section provides you with a list of major indexing & abstracting services. That is to say, each service began covering this periodical during the year noted in the right column. Most Websites which are listed below have indicated that they will either post, disseminate, compile, archive, cite or alert their own Website users with research-based content from this work. (This list is as current as the copyright date of this publication.)

Special Bibliographic Notes related to special journal issues (separates) and indexing/abstracting:

- indexing/abstracting services in this list will also cover material in any "separate" that is co-published simultaneously with Haworth's special thematic journal issue or DocuSerial. Indexing/abstracting usually covers material at the article/chapter level.
- monographic co-editions are intended for either non-subscribers or libraries which intend to purchase a second copy for their circulating collections.
- monographic co-editions are reported to all jobbers/wholesalers/approval plans. The source journal is listed as the "series" to assist the prevention of duplicate purchasing in the same manner utilized for books-in-series.
- to facilitate user/access services all indexing/abstracting services are encouraged to utilize the co-indexing entry note indicated at the bottom of the first page of each article/chapter/contribution.
- this is intended to assist a library user of any reference tool (whether print, electronic, online, or CD-ROM) to locate the monographic version if the library has purchased this version but not a subscription to the source journal.
- individual articles/chapters in any Haworth publication are also available through the Haworth Document Delivery Service (HDDS).

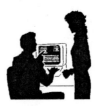

Promoting Civility
in Pharmacy Education

CONTENTS

ALL PHARMACEUTICAL PRODUCTS PRESS
BOOKS AND JOURNALS ARE PRINTED
ON CERTIFIED ACID-FREE PAPER

ABOUT THE EDITOR

Bruce A. Berger, Ph.D., R.Ph., is Professor and Head of Pharmacy Care Systems at Auburn University, where he was awarded an Alumni Professorship for his outstanding teaching, research, and service. His research interests include interpersonal and organizational communication and psychology and the application of these disciplines to the pharmacist's role in treatment adherence and treatment outcomes. He is also interested in developing new service roles for pharmacists. Dr. Berger has written or presented over 500 papers or seminars on these topics. He has attracted over two million dollars in funding to support his research and has been a project leader in a reengineering project for a major U.S. drug chain. Dr. Berger is the recipient of the Johnson & Johnson Award, the Lyman Award, and the first American Association of Colleges of Pharmacy's Award of Excellence for his research. He is the 2001 recipient of the Jack L. Beal Post Baccalaureate Alumni Award from Ohio State University. Dr. Berger writes a regular column in *US Pharmacist*. In 1997, he was named one of the 50 most influential people in U.S. pharmacy by *American Druggist*.

Introduction

Bruce A. Berger

This volume focuses on promoting civility in pharmacy education. While many in the academy have reported an increase in the incidence of incivilities in the classroom, the purpose of this work is not to debate whether this is true. The goal of this book is to describe the concerns involved and to provide realistic and practical solutions to the problems pharmacy educators face in a number of educational settings. And, as Kathy Franklin, an assistant professor of higher education at the University of Arkansas, says, "Historically, what's happening today isn't unusual. Are students today different from students ten years ago? Probably, because of demographic changes, consumerism, K-12 experiences. But is this a new trend? No" (1). Students today prefer self-directed learning, dislike close supervision, are cynical, tend to be less respectful or in awe of authority figures/faculty, desire immediate feedback, and like faculty who get to the point (2). What is especially different is that professors are held in lower esteem today, and this seems particularly insulting to many academics. Many professors "retaliate" with equally insulting behavior (1). As a result, incivilities often escalate, or the learning environment is destroyed or is greatly compromised.

This collection will explore promoting civility in several pharmacy education contexts. Brian Crabtree from the University of Mississippi

Bruce A. Berger, Ph.D., R.Ph., is Professor of Pharmacy Care Systems, Auburn University School of Pharmacy, 128 Miller Hall, Auburn University, AL 36849-5506 (E-mail: bergeba@auburn.edu).

[Haworth co-indexing entry note]: "Introduction." Berger, Bruce A. Co-published simultaneously in *Journal of Pharmacy Teaching* (Pharmaceutical Products Press, an imprint of The Haworth Press, Inc.) Vol. 9, No. 3, 2002, pp. 1-10; and: *Promoting Civility in Pharmacy Education* (ed: Bruce A. Berger) Pharmaceutical Products Press, an imprint of The Haworth Press, Inc., 2003, pp. 1-10. Single or multiple copies of this article are available for a fee from The Haworth Document Delivery Service [1-800-HAWORTH, 9:00 a.m. - 5:00 p.m. (EST). E-mail address: docdelivery@haworthpress.com].

http://www.haworthpress.com/store/product.asp?sku=J060
© 2003 by The Haworth Press, Inc. All rights reserved.
10.1300/J060v09n03_01

will discuss promoting civility in small classroom or small group settings. Diane Beck from Auburn University examines promoting civility in clinical settings. Holly Mason of Purdue University writes about civility in graduate education, while Dana Hammer from the University of Colorado discusses the relationship between professionalism and civility. Donna West from the University of Arkansas explores civility issues for new faculty members. Heidi Anderson-Harper of the University of Kentucky examines boundary violations and civility. I will discuss managing and promoting civility in large classrooms.

WHAT ARE INCIVILITIES?

Generally speaking, an incivility is a speech or action that is disrespectful or rude (3). At the American Association of Colleges of Pharmacy's Annual Meeting Teacher's Seminar in 2000, pharmacy educators were asked to identify incivilities. Appendix A summarizes their responses. In discussing what constitutes an incivility, as one might suspect, faculty did not all agree that certain behaviors were uncivil. For example, some faculty felt strongly that a student walking into class late was uncivil or rude, while many others said it did not bother them. Some faculty actually left the last row of the classroom open so that students coming in late could sit there without disrupting others. The important point that came out of this was that while faculty cannot always come to consensus on what constitutes uncivil behavior, faculty have a right (and an obligation) to make clear to students what kinds of behaviors they consider appropriate or inappropriate. In addition, students identified faculty sarcasm or public embarrassment of students (particularly when students ask questions in class) as the most annoying and frustrating uncivil behavior perpetrated by faculty. Each author will describe appropriate ways to prevent and manage incivilities in the educational environments they describe.

WHY DO INCIVILITIES OCCUR?

Appendix B summarizes faculty responses at the American Association of Colleges of Pharmacy's Annual Meeting Teacher's Seminar in 2000. The question posed was, "Why do incivilities occur?" While the list of incivilities by faculty and students is varied, with few exceptions, several items stand out. First, almost all of the incivilities listed can potentially be prevented or eliminated. We may not be able to do much about faculty pay raises, but answering students' questions respectfully is certainly doable and warranted. Coming prepared to class is not only doable but an obligation of professors to students. It should be noted that the focus of this series of articles will be on what we, as faculty, can do to prevent and appropriately respond to incivilities in various educational settings. Changing our own behavior will be far more productive than trying to change our students' behavior. This does not mean that we should not set limits or boundaries. We should. It will simply be far more useful to evaluate our own attitudes and actions in trying to prevent or respond to incivilities.

Secondly, incivilities occur far more often when people are stressed. For students, this often happens right before a major exam. When people experience fairly high levels of stress, they are far less likely to be tolerant, compassionate, and patient. Sensitivity to these levels of stress on the part of faculty (and students) will go a long way toward alleviating some problems. This does not imply that faculty should ignore incivilities because students are stressed; it simply means that in formulating a response, compassion, patience, and understanding will be far more effective than a punitive, equally disrespectful response.

An example may help. I require a paper in my course. My syllabus clearly spells out font and margin requirements, minimum page length, and referencing requirements. In addition, students are told that one point will be deducted for each unique grammar and spelling error. A male student who had over 40 unique grammar and spelling errors on his paper literally burst into my office one day, without knocking, threw his paper on my desk, and said, "I didn't know that this was a f*cking English class!" He was obviously very distressed . . . and uncivil.

While many faculty would have supported me if I had "thrown the little SOB out," this would have had many negative consequences. The student would have gone to his classmates, and what they would have heard about was how I disrespectfully threw him out. I teach a communication class, and it certainly would not appear to be that I was practicing what I preached. In addition, if I had said something like, "You are not going to talk to me that way. Now get out of my office!" it is highly unlikely that he would have ever reflected on his own behavior. This is an especially important point regarding dealing with incivilities or rude or disrespectful behavior. Often when people are the target of uncivil behavior, they somehow believe that they have the right to be uncivil in return. However, this only serves to escalate the problem and ensures that very little reflection takes place.

Using effective listening skills and setting appropriate boundaries increases the probability that the problem will not escalate and something may be learned. In this case, I looked at the student and said quietly, "You are obviously very angry and upset about your grade and I want to talk to you about that. However, I don't want to be yelled at and I don't want to be sworn at. If you can talk to me without yelling and swearing, we can do so now, otherwise, you will need to leave until you are ready to do so. What would you like to do?" The student turned red. His embarrassment was an indication to me that he actually caught himself behaving badly. I don't think this would have happened if I had yelled back. I honestly did not feel angry because I did not believe I had done anything wrong. In addition, I could see how stressed he was by the low grade he received. Nonetheless, a boundary needed to be set to clearly identify what behaviors I would and would not tolerate. Heidi Anderson-Harper will talk more about boundary violations in her section.

Incivilities also occur more often when there are unrealistic expectations on the part of faculty and students. Let's first look at unrealistic expectations that faculty may have of students. While it would be a wonderful world if students were always attentive, were always respectful, were in awe of my expertise, would obey my authority and my rules without question (or forgetting), and would not have emotional outbursts on occasion, anyone who has taught for even the shortest length of time knows that this world doesn't exist. Faculty who hold expectations of students that are unrealistic are often seen as punitive and uncaring in the classroom. When these expectations are not met, faculty blame students rather than adjusting expectations. Again, adjusting expectations does not mean that outbursts should be permitted; it means that they are handled with civility rather than disrespect.

Faculty sometimes inaccurately assess students' prior knowledge as students enter a new course. This results in classroom sessions and assignments that are either pitched too high or too low, resulting in frustration for both faculty and students. While it is legitimate to hold students accountable for previous course learning and materials, it is probably unrealistic to expect instant recall or recall of information that was taught but never mastered as a result of lacking assessment methods. It is vitally important, therefore, to assess students' prior knowledge when a new class begins, especially if previous course material is prerequisite learning.

Students also have irrational beliefs. Some believe that classes should be fun and exciting all of the time, that exams should be "easy," and that professors should be available at the whim of the student. In fact, some students believe that as "consumers" of education, they are owed these things. In addition, they believe that they should decide what is important, that they should decide how the class should be conducted, and that the professor works for them—*not* the university. A recent trend involves the student as a consumer or customer. The assumption here is that students are paying for a product–a degree; therefore, they are in the best position to know what they want and to decide whether the education they are getting is relevant and worthwhile. "The student-customer model seduces students into believing that they know what is best for them" (4). This consumerist model fails on a number of counts. First, a customer purchase does not obligate one to be accountable to the public. Yet, pharmacists are precisely that once they are conferred a degree and pass the board exams. Unlike a consumer scenario, paying for a degree (the product) does not entitle the student to getting one. The consumer model also assumes that the consumer is already knowledgeable about the product. That is certainly not true of students.

The mentality of this model creates problems in the classroom at numerous levels. Students believe that they are owed something. This may lend itself to uncivil behavior. Students will pressure faculty to satisfy the "consumer" and thus lower standards. It allows students to believe that they have a right to pressure faculty for better grades and, in general, promotes an antischolarly approach to higher education (4). The important point here is that students are *not* consumers and faculty need not "cave in" to this mentality and lower their standards to please students.

Lastly, powerlessness seems to breed incivility. When students feel powerless or when faculty do not feel supported for any number of reasons, some form of aggressive or passive-aggressive behavior often follows to make up for this feeling of powerlessness. Frequent input and feedback are antidotes to this kind of powerlessness, in addition to support of faculty by administrators.

CHARACTERISTICS OF FACULTY WITH FEWER INCIDENTS OF INCIVILITIES IN THE CLASSROOM

While we are often quick to point a finger at students and say that they are "less respectful than they used to be," Boice concluded the following as a result of a study on classroom incivilities (CI):

> Clearly teachers were the most crucial initiators of CI. And, as a rule, their most telling provocations occurred during the first few days of courses. Conversely, professors who most consistently displayed immediacies and positive motivators were least involved in incidents of CI, their own or their students'. (5)

What this means is teachers have a great deal of influence on whether incivilities occur in their classrooms. In fact, research confirms that a much higher frequency of incivilities by students occur in classrooms where the teacher has been uncivil or does not establish appropriate boundaries or guidelines right away (5).

More incivilities occur in classrooms with teachers who are less competent and less immediate in their behaviors. Competence refers to awareness and engaging in prosocial behaviors. Boice reports:

> Students decide to resist and misbehave depending largely on two interrelated kinds of teacher behaviors. One is a matter of whether the teacher employs mostly prosocial motivators (e.g., "Do you understand?" and "You can do better") or antisocial motivators (e.g., threats and guilt induction). The second is about immediacy–the extent to which the teacher gives off verbal and nonverbal signs of warmth, friendliness, and liking (e.g., forward leans, smiles, purposeful gestures, eye contact). With positive motivators and particularly, immediacy, student inclinations to CI drop off dramatically. But without these skills, teachers are seen as cold, uncaring, and incompetent by their students–as deserving of incivilities. (5)

Other low immediacy behaviors included fast-paced, noninvolving lectures; low or no involvement outside of class; ill-defined or no office hours (or office hours not honored or kept); statements indicating that they do not wish to be bothered outside of class; discouraging questions in class or in some way embarrassing or putting down the questioner (being funny or sarcastic at the student's expense). Power and respect in the classroom is relational. Development of the teacher-student relationship is critical to deterring or decreasing incivilities. More on this subject will be covered in each educational setting.

One last point needs to be made in this section. If we, as faculty, are to be as effective as possible in developing civil behaviors in our students, we must be role models–mentors. Being the students' friends or parents does not work, and quite frankly, it is inappropriate. Some junior faculty members make the mistake of trying to befriend students. Students do not need us to be their friends. They don't need faculty drinking buddies. They need mentors. Mentors model the desired attitudes and behaviors. Mentors care deeply about their protégés. Mentors simply respect and maintain the necessary boundaries in the professional-client relationship. Without these boundaries, confusion exists in the relationship.

> Boundaries are limits that allow for a safe connection based on the client's needs. When these limits are altered, what is allowed in the relationship becomes ambiguous. Such ambiguity is often expressed as an intrusion into the sphere of safety. The pain of a violation is frequently delayed, and the violation itself may not be recognized or felt until harmful sequences emerge. (6)

We are entrusted with a great deal of power by our students because of our expertise. As a result, they are put in a very vulnerable place. We are entrusted to put their needs ahead of ours. Boundary violations are acts that breach the core intent of the professional-client relationship and, as a result, violate or destroy safety. Befriending the very students we are evaluating and mentoring confuses the boundary.

Finally, faculty must realize that we are "on" all of the time. Our behavior is being constantly monitored by students whether we like it or not. We must become aware of our own attitudes and behaviors if we are to effectively model the attitudes and behaviors we desire.

EMOTIONAL IMPACT

It is unfortunate that when people discuss incivilities very rarely do they talk about the emotional impact. Generally, they discuss what happened and ascribe blame. It is rare when people talk about what happened emotionally, yet it is the emotional impact of incivilities that can often disrupt a student's desire to learn or a faculty member's desire to teach. When the learning environment becomes unsafe or threatened due to an incivility or repeated incivilities, the student's education always suffers. Appendix C summarizes faculty responses on the emotional impact of incivilities. The emotional impact of an incivility can be devastating. Incivilities can cause professors to lose self-esteem and self-confidence in their teaching, lose self-confidence in their research efforts, abandon teaching, become indifferent in the classroom, and fear for their safety (this is especially true for female faculty). Incivilities can cause students to become increasingly uninvolved in a course, become increasingly hostile in the classroom, fear for their safety (this is especially true when boundaries are violated–more on this later), and lose their desire to learn (6).

SUMMARY

Incivilities are often difficult to cope with in an educational environment. They can disrupt learning and have a lasting emotional impact on both students and faculty. It is our hope that this book will provide you with ways to promote civility and to prevent and manage incivilities in different educational settings within pharmacy.

REFERENCES

1. Schneider A. Insubordination and intimidation signals the end of decorum in many classrooms. *Chron Higher Educ.* 1998; (Mar 27):A1-A14. Available at http://chronicle.com/colloquy/98/rude/background.htm.

2. Little L. Leading four generations. *Acad Leader.* 2000; (Mar):5-7.

3. Teaching Resources Center, College of Arts and Sciences, Indiana University. Available at http://www.indiana.edu/~teaching.

4. Albanese M. Students are not customers: A better model for medical education. *Acad Med.* 1999; 74:1172-86.

5. Boice B. Classroom incivilities. *Res Higher Educ.* 1996; 37:453-86.

6. Peterson MR. At personal risk: Boundary violations in professional-client relationships. New York: W. W. Norton & Co.; 1992.

APPENDIX A. What Are Incivilities?

- Several types
- Student to faculty
  - Faculty to student
  - Student to administration
  - Student to student
  - Faculty to faculty
  - Faculty to administration
  - Administration to faculty
- Anything that distracts from learning
- Cell phones, computers
- Lack of confidentiality
- Sexual harassment
- Cheating
- Breaking rules
  - Food in class
  - Newspapers, littering
- Demeaning, condescending behavior/attitudes
- Locking doors to keep out latecomers
- Sarcastic remarks by students and/or faculty
- Abusing a learning disability
- Not taking appropriate responsibility
- Electronic incivility–bulletin boards, e-mails, the actual message content
- Cultural, generational differences in values

KEEP IN MIND, WHAT ONE CONSIDERS TO BE UNCIVIL BEHAVIOR (WALKING IN LATE TO CLASS), ANOTHER MIGHT FIND PERFECTLY ACCEPTABLE OR TOLERABLE. FACULTY HAVE THE RIGHT TO EXPRESS, UP FRONT, WHAT THEY CONSIDER TO BE INAPPROPRIATE BEHAVIOR IN THEIR CLASSES. REASONS SHOULD BE PROVIDED.

APPENDIX B. Why Do Incivilities Occur?

- Students
  - Lack of respect for others
  - Needs of student not met or not met with dignity
  - No clear expectations given
  - Inappropriate "role model" as instructor
  - Poor communication by instructor
  - Lack of fairness
  - No energy from instructor
  - Outdated materials
  - Lack of respect by instructor
  - Not enough feedback
  - Material covered and tests are incongruent

- ○ Don't understand relevance of material
- ○ Entitlement mentality–the student as consumer
- ○ Lack of power by student or inappropriate use of power by faculty
- ○ Boundary violations
- ○ Lack of preparation by faculty
- ○ Faculty arrive late and/or ends too early or too late
- ○ Instructor's attitude (arrogance, indifference, etc.)
- ○ Inconsistency in expectations from one faculty member to another
- ○ Faculty allow incivilities to occur . . . don't say anything, ignore
- ○ Personal problems
- ○ Work
- ○ Faculty member is unapproachable
- ○ Lack of dialog

- Faculty
  - ○ Overworked, underpaid, lack of resources
  - ○ Poor attitudes by students
  - ○ Frustration, stress
  - ○ Students come to class unprepared
  - ○ Unrealistic or inconsistent expectations
  - ○ Student lack of understanding about patient care
  - ○ Lack of reward for teaching
  - ○ Personal problems
  - ○ Different goals, standards, values than students
  - ○ CHAOS!
  - ○ Boundary violations

APPENDIX C. Emotional Impact of Incivilities on Faculty and Students.

- Anger
- Frustration
- Apathy–withdrawal–depression
- Insecurity
- Helplessness
- Fear–threat
- Poor performance
- Manipulated
- Intimidated
- Dread (of going to class, of teaching the class)
- Defensiveness–isolation, victimization
- Hostile environment
- Grapevine–rumors about the class

INCIVILITIES CAN BE DEVASTATING TO FACULTY AND STUDENTS. THEY CAN RUIN CAREERS OR INJURE SELF-CONFIDENCE AND CAUSE DESPOND-ENCE. THEY ARE TO BE TAKEN SERIOUSLY.

Promoting Civility in Large Classrooms

Bruce A. Berger

INTRODUCTION

The large classroom is often a venue where more incivilities occur because students can hide among the masses. The ability to be anonymous often produces attitudes and behaviors that are less than respectful, especially if these attitudes and behaviors are encouraged by other students. In addition, because large classroom are sometimes very impersonal, incivilities are more likely to occur. When people (either students or professors) are seen as objects, they are no longer human, caring, or capable of being harmed by someone else's words or actions. As such, they are more likely to be subjected to incivilities. This is consistent with Boice's research stating that faculty who have more incivilities inflicted on them are often seen as distant, cold, less competent, and less immediate in their behaviors (1). This information should provide faculty with insight on how to reduce incivilities in the large classroom, that is, be seen as human, caring, and competent.

This manuscript examines how to promote civility in the large classroom setting. It examines the kinds of incivilities that occur and how to take preventive measures and respond appropriately when incivilities do occur.

Bruce A. Berger, Ph.D., R.Ph., is Professor of Pharmacy Care Systems, Auburn University School of Pharmacy, 128 Miller Hall, Auburn University, AL 36849-5506 (E-mail: bergeba@auburn.edu).

Reprinted with the permission from *American Journal of Pharmaceutical Education* 2000;64:445-50.

[Haworth co-indexing entry note]: "Promoting Civility in Large Classrooms." Berger, Bruce A. Co-published simultaneously in *Journal of Pharmacy Teaching* (Pharmaceutical Products Press, an imprint of The Haworth Press, Inc.) Vol. 9, No. 3, 2002, pp. 11-22; and: *Promoting Civility in Pharmacy Education* (ed: Bruce A. Berger) Pharmaceutical Products Press, an imprint of The Haworth Press, Inc., 2003, pp. 11-22. Single or multiple copies of this article are available for a fee from The Haworth Document Delivery Service [1-800-HAWORTH, 9:00 a.m. - 5:00 p.m. (EST). E-mail address: docdelivery@haworthpress.com].

http://www.haworthpress.com/store/product.asp?sku=J060
10.1300/J060v09n03_02

CAUSES OF INCIVILITIES

While we are often quick to point a finger at students and say that they are "less respectful than they used to be," Boice concluded as a result of a study on classroom incivilities (CI): "Clearly teachers were the most crucial initiators of CI. And, as a rule, their most telling provocations occurred during the first few days of courses. Conversely, professors who most consistently displayed immediacies and positive motivators were least involved in incidents of CI, their own or their students'" (2). What this means is that teachers have a great deal of influence on whether incivilities occur in their classrooms. More on this later.

In addition to the above, it is obvious to many that students will engage in uncivil behaviors in and out of the classroom. Specifically, the following beliefs, attitudes, or behaviors on the part of faculty and students are likely to contribute to or increase the rate of incivilities (3):

- Students are annoyed by:
  - Lateness–on the part of students and faculty
  - Early or late stopping of class
  - Cutting or canceling of class
  - Loud, disruptive talking by other students in the classroom. Unless told otherwise, students *expect* faculty to take immediate action about disruptions in the classroom.
  - Rude comments/gestures (creates both annoyance and uncomfortableness/fear) by *both* students and faculty.
- Students are more likely to exhibit incivilities before or after major exams or projects.
- Distrust of professors:
  - Those who display less immediate and caring behaviors.
  - Via surprise quizzes, tests, and/or exam items. Planned quizzes are acceptable as long they are part of announced examinations, projects, etc., in the syllabus.

TYPES OF INCIVILITY

There are primarily two types of incivilities; passive and active. *Passive* incivility includes inattention, lateness, mild disruptions (shuffling papers, notebooks, or backpacks; wearing a headset; talking on a cell phone; walking in and out of the class; etc.). It also includes not completing the necessary work, asking for extensions, and making excuses. *Overt or active* incivilities include direct challenges to the teacher in a nonrespectful manner, vulgar language/gestures to teacher, insulting comments or actions to other students, and physical threats.

To Address Passive Incivilities

1. Make direct eye contact with the student(s) involved. Stop talking and don't start until they're with you again and notice that you are looking at them.
2. Move to that part of the class and direct a question to someone next to the student talking.
3. Get students actively involved in the classroom. Don't lecture continuously without asking questions or assigning small tasks. Use in-class small group exercises for brief (15 minutes) amounts of time to change the pace in the classroom and get more students involved in the discussion. Also assign outside small group activities that involve the course materials. Use the "lecture" time to have students report group findings. To keep this activity from being repetitive and tedious, have groups only add new information from the previous groups' reports.
4. Speak to students privately about their actions. This means out of the sight and hearing of other students. State specifically what happened, how you felt, and what you want in the future ("I have noticed you talking several times in class over the past few days. If you have questions about the material or are confused, by all means, please ask. Otherwise, I would appreciate it if you make sure this doesn't happen again. It is hard for me to conduct a class without distractions. Having them makes it even harder."). Do not make this a personal attack (Your talking in class is disrespectful and completely unprofessional. It better not happen again!). Simply state what happened and what you now expect.
5. Ask, don't accuse. Make it a friendly conversation to find out what is wrong ("I noticed that you were talking in class a few times today. Is there something I can help with that is causing concern or confusion?").

To Address Overt or Active Incivilities

1. Listen respectfully to student complaints–don't become defensive. Reflect back your understanding of the problem and sort is-

sues, when necessary. Talk with the student(s) privately, but not in an isolated place. Keep in mind that just because others may treat you disrespectfully does not mean that you now have the right to do so in return. People are going to go crazy now and then . . . don't go with them! Remember, we need to stay in our mentoring role as much as possible. This means meeting disrespect with appropriate responses. For example, during class you are going over an exam and a student says, "This is ridiculous! This test was so tricky! I don't know why I even bothered studying." If you sense that this is a common concern, you may want to address it (especially if you use item analyses) and listen carefully to which questions seem to be a problem and why. This may help you write better questions, learn where problem areas exist with the material, or help you decide that some questions are confusing and may need to be discarded. If this is an isolated instance, simply tell the student you would like to talk to him or her about specific concerns after class. When class ends, ask for specific examples and simply explain your justification for the test item. If the student makes a good point, acknowledge it. However, if the student behaves rudely, simply state, "I know you are upset and angry about some of these test items and I want to discuss them with you and learn why you are upset. However, I want to be treated with respect. This means no yelling. If you can do this, we will continue, otherwise, this conversation is over until you can. What would you like to do?"

2. Reassure the rest of the class. If an incident should occur in the class in which a student is uncivil and leaves, it is important to reassure the class that you will not allow their learning environment to be disrupted. If you have behaved badly (yes, every now and then we lose it), apologize and assure them it won't happen again.

3. Be honest when something is not working. For example, you have tried a new exercise in the class, and it has bombed. Say something like, "I can tell by your responses that this is not going as well as I had hoped. How could I have done this differently?" Welcome their constructive suggestions and thank them. This could actually be an opportunity to promote a productive environment.

4. Know and use the chain of command in your school or on your campus. If you are having persistent problems with a student or students and have talked with them privately, to no avail, it is important to use the chain of command available in the school. If

there is no written procedure, it is extremely important that one be developed.

For Any Incivility

1. Don't ignore it, hoping it will go away–it won't. Everything you do in the classroom conveys meaning to the students. If you are a great teacher but allow talking and disruptions to continue, you are essentially condoning the behavior. This often creates disrespect in the classroom.
2. Don't laugh off inappropriate comments or behavior. Don't allow your need to be liked to get in the way of being confrontational when necessary. Talk to the individual after class or on a break and let him or her know how you feel about the behavior and what will be done if it continues in the future; for example, "Tom, I did not like the lewd (or sexist) comment you made in class. I was offended by it. In addition, that kind of language is a violation of the school's Honor Code. If it happens again, I will report you to the Honor Board." Permitting inappropriate comments and behavior simply sanctions them and sets the stage for more of the same.
3. Don't get in an argument, become defensive, or take it personally.
4. Don't press for immediate explanation of the offensive behavior. This will only serve to shame or embarrass the student in front of his peers and create more hostility.
5. Don't walk away from the student. Again, this is like ignoring the action, which sanctions it.
6. Don't make exceptions about assignments or for uncivil behavior. This sets you up for disrespect in the future.
7. Don't carry it all by yourself. Get advice. Talk to other (particularly, more senior) faculty for input.

PREVENTIVE MEASURES

- Make it clear in your syllabus what behaviors are not acceptable in your course. What are your expectations? Discuss these expectations on the first day of class. Also be clear about what will be done to "violators" (see Appendix A).
- Consider the development of an honor code (and honor board) at your school that defines violations as including uncivil behavior (see Appendix B). If nothing else, this should be an important

topic for faculty discussion. Often honor codes cover academic dishonesty but not professional (mis)conduct. In a professional school, it seems reasonable to identify appropriate and inappropriate behaviors.

- Reexamine your classroom. Some questions you should ask yourself (or your students) (3):

  ○ Is my classroom boring? Do I actively involve the students, or do I spend a lot of time "pontificating?" Can I take lecture material and make it more interactive using small group discussions, then debriefing?

  ○ Is the material covered necessary? Is the material I cover necessary to the students' mastery of the subject? If not, discard it. On the other hand, if the students can read it as well as I can say it, why not use lecture time to answer questions and take the material beyond the reading? Can't get them to read in advance? Give announced quizzes on the reading instead of midterm exams.

  ○ Am I aloof or defensive? Studies confirm that professors who are aloof, defensive, and not respectful to students have a higher amount of incivility in their classrooms.

  ○ Am I complacent about uncivil or disruptive behavior? Remember, doing nothing is consent.

  ○ Do I get feedback from students regularly throughout the quarter or semester to address or head off problems? This can be done by identifying three or four students in the class to meet with on a weekly basis to discuss how things are going, or an assessment can be done after each week's class meetings to see how students are doing (see Appendix C).

PERSONALIZING THE LARGE CLASSROOM

As stated previously, students behave in ways in a large classroom they never would behave in a small class. The impersonal nature of the class allows students to hide and often objectify the teacher (objectification reduces the teacher to an object–a thing that is more open to abuse). Engaging in more prosocial and verbally immediate behaviors is important in reducing objectification.

Solutions for large classrooms:

- *Weekly Workshops.* Many professors hold weekly workshop sessions that are not required. This is a good chance for students to review the material and get to know the teacher better. Moreover, they are less likely to behave uncivilly in a smaller group.
- *One-Minute Papers.* This is a voluntary exercise that is held at the last five to ten minutes of a class period. Class is stopped a few minutes early, and students are asked to write down any questions or problems they are having. Their papers are dropped in a box at the back of room. Several of the questions posed are addressed at the beginning of the next class period or answers are e-mailed to the whole class. The responsiveness to questions creates a cooperative climate. It encourages students to ask questions without risking embarrassment.
- *Student Interest.* Get to class early and mingle with the students. Get to know their names. Take an interest in them.
- *Weekly Evaluations.* These can be done each lecture or once a week and allow for frequent feedback so that small problems don't become large ones (see Appendix C for an example). Evaluations allow for feedback and responsiveness to build rapport. Also, give weekly quizzes to assess problems before they become big. I give a quiz for each set of readings. Students are allowed to ask as many questions as they want before the quiz. Then they take a 15-minute quiz (15 multiple choice, true-false, matching questions). We go over the quiz immediately after they take it. The quizzes and the process have several benefits:

  - Students actually read the material before class. This has increased the quality of the classroom discussions tremendously and has allowed for greater participation and interaction.
  - Because students keep up with the readings, they don't have to "cram" for the final exam.
  - Students get immediate feedback about how they did. In addition, because we go over the quiz immediately, I get immediate feedback about possible confusion and problem areas. In addition, I use items analyses to detect problems with subject matter and/or framing of questions.
  - Discussing the quiz material is a natural lead-in to the discussion topic(s) for the day. Quiz discussions are a great opportunity to discuss why answers are both correct and incorrect and draw upon the reading.

SUMMARY

Promoting civility in a large classroom setting takes planning, work, and introspection. Planning reduces the chance that an incivility will occur by letting students know what you expect up front. In addition, planning allows you to make your classes more interactive by building in small group work and extra sessions. This will also help make your classes more personal, along with arriving to class early and getting to know the students in your classes. All of this takes hard work and dedication to teaching. Finally, introspection is needed to really evaluate whether you are doing all you can to make your classes more interesting and personal. Small, but sustained efforts lead to vast improvement in large classroom settings.

REFERENCES

1. Boice B. Classroom incivilities. *Res Higher Educ*. 1996; 37:453-86.

2. Teaching Resources Center, College of Arts and Sciences, Indiana University. Available at http://www.indiana.edu/~teaching.

3. Berger BA. Incivility. *Am J Pharm Educ*. 2000; 64:445-50.

4. Schneider A. Insubordination and intimidation signals the end of decorum in many classrooms. *Chron Higher Educ*. 1998; (Mar 27):A1-A14. Available at http://chronicle.com/colloquy/98/rude/background.htm.

5. Carbone E. Students behaving badly in large classes. *N Directions Teach Learn*. 1999; 77(Spr):35-43.

APPENDIX A

Classroom Demeanor: An Excerpt from One Syllabus–Example 1

It is your responsibility to attend class. If you miss a class meeting for any reason, you will be held responsible for all material covered and announcements made in your absence. . . .

Lecture attendance is neither required nor noted. However, BE ON TIME AND REMAIN FOR THE ENTIRE PERIOD OR DO NOT COME AT ALL. This class is too large to have people crawling over each other or standing in front of the projector while trying to find a seat or leaving after the lecture has begun. Arriving late and/or leaving early is inconsiderate of your colleagues.

This class is also too large for chit-chat, please do not. You are unaware of how far your voices carry in FAV 150 and how disturbing it is to your classmates to be forced to endure your idle chatter and giggling. The students who sit near you are not interested in your romantic lives, how out-of-touch you think your parents are, how stupid you think your teachers are, etc. You may not realize how disturbing your "private" conversations are when others are trying to listen to a lecture. . . .

Everyone who registers for this class is an adult. You are legally able to marry without parental consent, buy a home, pay taxes, vote, work, budget your money, defend your country in military service, etc. You should also be adult enough not to disturb others. Mindless talking during class is immature, inconsiderate behavior. Please ask questions or make comments about the art work that will benefit the entire class, but leave the chit-chat in the halls where it belongs.

–From a course syllabus by Professor Susanne J. Warma, Utah State U.

Classroom Demeanor: An Excerpt from One Syllabus–Example 2

The course policy on class attendance and excused absences is the same as that described in the Auburn University Student Handbook. Arrangements to make up missed work (assignments or exams) due to excused absences will be initiated by the student. Only students presenting an excused absence will be allowed to make up any missed work. These assignments must be made up within one week following the date the assignment was due. Otherwise, missed work will be assigned a grade of zero.

Students will be allowed to make up any missed exams only if the instructor is notified in advance. Such absences must be for legitimate, documented purposes as indicated in the Handbook. The make-up exam will most likely be a different form of the exam. No student will be allowed to take an exam prior to its scheduled time.

Cheating, unprofessional behavior, and incivility in the classroom are all considered to be violations of the Auburn University School of Pharmacy Code of Ethical and Professional Conduct. The instructor will not hesitate to report violators of the Code to the Honor Board. It is your responsibility to be knowledgeable of the Code and what constitutes violations.

APPENDIX B. Excerpts from the Auburn University School of Pharmacy Code of Ethical and Professional Conduct.

3.00 **VIOLATIONS**

3.01 Violations of the School of Pharmacy Code of Ethical and Professional Conduct pertaining to academic honesty **include but are not limited to**:

3.01.1 The receipt, possession or use of any material or assistance not authorized by the instructor in the preparation of papers, reports, examinations, or any class assignment to be submitted for credit as a part of a course or to be submitted to fulfill School of Pharmacy requirements. The receipt, possession or use of any aid or material prohibited by the instructor while an examination or quiz is in progress.

3.01.2 Knowingly giving assistance not authorized by the instructor to another in the preparation of papers, reports, or laboratory data and products.

3.01.3 Knowingly giving assistance not authorized by the instructor to another while an examination or quiz is in progress.

3.01.4 Lending, giving, selling or otherwise furnishing to another any material or information not authorized by the instructor which can be shown to contain the questions or answers to any examination or quiz scheduled to be given at a subsequent date.

3.01.5 The submission of papers, reports, projects or similar course requirements, or parts thereof, that is not the work of the student submitting them. Also, the use of direct quotations or ideas of another in materials to be submitted for credit without appropriate acknowledgment.

3.01.6 Knowingly submitting a paper, report, examination or any class assignment that has been altered or corrected, in part or in whole, for reevaluation or regarding.

3.01.7 Altering or attempting to alter an assigned grade on any official School of Pharmacy or University record.

3.01.8 The instructor may delineate in advance other actions he/she considers to be a violation of the Code.

3.02 Violations of the School of Pharmacy Code of Professional Conduct pertaining to professional conduct include:

3.02.1 Purposely falsifying applications, forms or records prior to admission to the School of Pharmacy, or while enrolled in the School's professional programs.

3.02.2 Knowingly producing false evidence (or rumors) against another or providing false statements or charges in bad faith against another. Knowingly publishing or circulating false information concerning any member of the University faculty, student body, staff or community.

3.02.3 Contributing to, or engaging in, any activity which disrupts or obstructs the teaching, research or extension programs of the School of Pharmacy or University, either on the campus or at affiliated training sites.

3.02.4 Threatening or purposely committing physical violence against any member of the University faculty, student body, staff, or community.

3.02.5 Misusing or misrepresenting one's status as a Pharmacy student or the right to use any University property and facilities.

3.02.6 Stealing, damaging, defacing, or unauthorized use of any property of the School of Pharmacy or University. Diversion of any School of Pharmacy or University property to one's own use.

3.02.7 Engaging in any facet of Pharmacy practice prior to graduation unless under the direct supervision of a licensed practitioner or otherwise allowed by law.

3.02.8 Intentionally revealing the names of the charging party, the accused, witnesses or the facts involved in an alleged violation except in accordance with the provisions of this Code, or revealing the confidential proceedings of an Honor Board hearing.

3.02.9 Failure to report known violations of the School of Pharmacy Code of Ethical and Professional Conduct.

3.02.10 Use, possession, or participating in the trafficking of illegal drugs or substances.

3.02.11 Unauthorized accessing of information about faculty, staff, or students of the School of Pharmacy, or patients/clients, that is private or confidential.

3.02.12 Unauthorized revealing of information about faculty, staff, or students of the School of Pharmacy, or patients/clients, that is private or confidential.

APPENDIX C. Weekly Class Assessment Form.

===

Teacher's Name_____   Date _____

TOPIC_____

Please circle the number that describes your response to each statement below, according to this scale:

Strongly Agree 5	Agree 4	Not Applicable or Neutral 3	Disagree 2	Strongly Disagree 1

		5	4	3	2	1
1.	I learned something today I didn't know.	5	4	3	2	1
2.	I enjoyed today's session.	5	4	3	2	1
3.	The information presented was useful to me.	5	4	3	2	1
4.	The speaker was knowledgeable on the subject.	5	4	3	2	1
5.	The speaker was interesting to listen to.	5	4	3	2	1
6.	The speaker encouraged questions.	5	4	3	2	1
7.	The speaker answered the questions respectfully.	5	4	3	2	1

COMMENTS ABOUT THIS SESSION OR THE COURSE:

At midterm, ask students to write answers to the following questions.
1) What do you like about this course?
2) What do you dislike? What needs improvements and how would you improve it?

Collate the answers and send a copy to each student by e-mail or pass it out.

Promoting Civility in the Small Classroom or Small Group Setting

INTRODUCTION

Incidents of incivility in higher education have always occurred. Although not quantified by well-designed research, a widely held perception in pharmacy education as well as higher education in general–indeed, among society–is that incivility is increasing. Organ lamented an emerging incivility at surgical society meetings (1). He describes civility as "synonymous with courtesy, politeness . . . the avoidance of rudeness." An interesting study by Lashley and Meneses evaluated incivility among nursing education programs (2). Yelling or verbal abuse toward instructors or peers was reported by 66% and 53% of study respondents, respectively. Twenty-five percent of respondents reported objectionable physical contact by a student to an instructor.

Relatively little has been published on this topic that relates specifically to pharmacy education. Bruce Berger's presentation at the AACP Annual Meeting Teacher's Seminar in 2000 and subsequent paper, as well as this collection, are among the few major commentaries on this topic in pharmacy education (3). Precise quantitative studies are lack-

Brian L. Crabtree, Pharm.D., is in the Department of Pharmacy Practice, School of Pharmacy, University of Mississippi Medical Center, 2500 North State Street, Jackson, MS 39216-4505 (E-mail: bcrabtre@netdoor.com).

[Haworth co-indexing entry note]: "Promoting Civility in the Small Classroom or Small Group Setting." Crabtree, Brian L. Co-published simultaneously in *Journal of Pharmacy Teaching* (Pharmaceutical Products Press, an imprint of The Haworth Press, Inc.) Vol. 9, No. 3, 2002, pp. 23-36; and: *Promoting Civility in Pharmacy Education* (ed: Bruce A. Berger) Pharmaceutical Products Press, an imprint of The Haworth Press, Inc., 2003, pp. 23-36. Single or multiple copies of this article are available for a fee from The Haworth Document Delivery Service [1-800-HAWORTH, 9:00 a.m. - 5:00 p.m. (EST). E-mail address: docdelivery@haworthpress.com].

http://www.haworthpress.com/store/product.asp?sku=J060
© 2003 by The Haworth Press, Inc. All rights reserved.
10.1300/J060v09n03_03

ing. Formal conferences and informal networking among faculty appear to indicate a consensus that incidents of incivility are increasing. Dr. Berger's introduction in this issue summarizes various types of incivilities that may occur, most often in large classroom settings, but also in a variety of other settings.

Most literature focuses on incivilities in a traditional classroom or in one-to-one interpersonal interactions outside the classroom. Little or no literature has addressed the small group learning environment. The small group environment has become more important in recent years as the academy and accreditation standards have emphasized active, self-directed learning strategies, with students working in teams and using faculty members more as tutors and resources rather than simply as conduits of factual information.

TYPES OF INCIVILITIES

Certain incivilities are common to both the large classroom and the small group classroom. Missing class, arriving late, not preparing for class, making rude comments, and exhibiting other behaviors may occur in either setting. Some incidents, however, are more likely to occur in one setting or the other. In the large classroom, it is possible for students to be more "anonymous" than in the small classroom. In small group settings, particularly in groups of less than ten students, it is not possible for students to "hide" and remain anonymous. Additionally, small group classes typically involve greater collaboration and group work than large classes. Each student has a greater responsibility to the others to stay current, to be prepared, and to carry a "share of the load." Lack of preparedness harms not only the poorly prepared student, but all others in the group who depend on their peers in the learning process. With a vertical integration of academic classroom disciplines and a decrease in lecture-based instruction, such incivilities may be more likely to occur.

As Dr. Berger has discussed, incivility is more likely to occur during periods of stress. Students often feel greater scrutiny in small groups, both by the teacher or facilitator and their peers. For many students, this is not a problem and brings out their natural interpersonal skills. For others, particularly students who are naturally shy or reserved, functioning in a small group can cause performance-related stress similar to that experienced by many people when they are about to deliver a speech or musical recital. Combined with greater expectations of pre-

paredness, always having to be "on" in a small group can lead to incivilities. Particular examples include exasperated and inappropriate public
protests about the nature of the course. It is not uncommon to hear comments such as, "Why are we doing this? We're paying you to teach us,
not just sit here and ask us questions!" Students who are not fully prepared and affect the learning of others may find themselves the target of
incivilities from peers. "Look, if you don't pull your weight, you're going to get us all in trouble. Get with the program!" The author knows of
at least one instance in which such an exchange escalated into a physical
altercation in the restroom after class.

Another major stress-related issue that can lead to incivilities is the
type of performance assessment in a small group class. Since desired
performance encompasses considerably more than knowledge acquisition, students are assessed by different methods and instruments than
those to which they are accustomed. For example, the shy student who
is assessed on the basis of quality and quantity of group participation
may feel discriminated against on the basis of personality traits. Such a
student may become angry toward the facilitator when this aspect of the
grade is low. Other measurements may reflect performance on standards such as use of appropriate learning resources, quality of writing
assignments, and depth and breadth of knowledge acquisition. Some
schools have adopted what has been termed "high stakes" systems of
assessment that require satisfactory performance on each measure without averaging of all measures. Such a system of increased scrutiny,
novel methods of assessment, higher stakes associated with assessment,
and nontraditional or unfamiliar faculty roles places the student under a
greater degree of stress. This is particularly true if course failure delays
progression toward the expected graduation date. As a result, students
who receive less than desired or less than accustomed grades in small
group classes are more likely to accuse a faculty member or the institution of improperly evaluating them or discriminating against them. At
one school, students have written anonymous messages about the course
director and posted them to internet sites or sent letters to university administrators accusing the instructor of improper behavior, circumvent-
ing the usual administrative channels.

The converse of the shy and/or stressed student in a small group class
is the outgoing and glib student who can dominate the group. Such a
student can inhibit other students from participating fully, sometimes
even cutting off discussion before another student is finished. Other students, especially more reserved or shy students, simply retreat and become even more passive. When a group has multiple strong and outgoing

personalities, the potential exists to antagonize each other. They may fear that their grade may suffer because they do not have free rein.

The faculty member who facilitates or directs a small group experience is perhaps the greatest influence on causing and preventing incidents of incivility. The familiarity of members of the group, including the facilitator, can lead to a breakdown in important barriers such as the faculty-student role or the mentor-mentee role. If the facilitator becomes merely another member of the group, known to the students on a first-name basis, socializing frequently with the students, then objective evaluation by the facilitator becomes more difficult. Students may have unrealistic expectations of how they will be evaluated because of the relationship. Conversely, the informality and closeness of a small group setting can enhance the learning relationship. If the facilitator is too distant or aloof, the opportunity to optimize learning is lost.

Another relationship issue between faculty members and students in small groups is unrealistic expectations of the facilitator. Facilitators who expect students to behave deferentially or in a subservient manner are more likely to inspire incivility. For example, if the facilitator makes statements such as, "I have more important things to do than sit in this group. I have patients to see in my clinic," then students feel devalued and are more likely to act out. Facilitators who set a class schedule then do not arrive on time, particularly when class is scheduled to meet very early or very late, thus committing an incivility themselves, are likely to cause anger and stress among students. Facilitators who ridicule students during a small group class have also been uncivil. An example could be laughing derisively at a student's comment or question or making a remark such as, "That was a dumb question!"

PREVENTION AND MANAGEMENT OF INCIVILITIES IN SMALL GROUPS

The old saying "an ounce of prevention is worth a pound of cure" could not be more true than when considering incivilities in small groups. Many of the points in Dr. Berger's introduction and prior article apply well to small group settings.

The course syllabus and orientation to the course are crucial. Students must understand the learning model and how it differs from traditional classroom learning. Differing roles, responsibilities, and obligations of both students and facilitators must be made clear. Behavioral standards must be made clear in advance and in writing. Performance standards and methods of assessment must be public documents. The role of the facilitator as a coach or tutor, not a transmitter of facts, should be clearly described. Once a detailed orientation is accomplished, facilitators must follow course policy and procedure uniformly for all groups and all students. Example topic areas of such an orientation are listed in Appendix A.

Appropriate professional boundaries between students and faculty must be preserved. In the small group setting more than in the large group setting, the facilitator functions as a mentor, a role model. A comfortable, safe learning environment depends on such a relationship. Facilitators must affirm students' learning and create an environment in which all contributions are welcome and valid. Ridicule or personal criticism is never warranted. Prosocial behaviors that affirm students and their learning will prevent most incivilities. Warmth, friendliness, evidence of concern, and availability all enhance a feeling of affirmation, empowerment in the learning process, and safety for the student.

Performance feedback needs to be repeated and sufficiently frequent that students know early in the experience how they are doing and have ample opportunities to improve and optimize their performance. This is particularly important when novel or innovative assessment methods or high stakes assessment is used. The student must feel that the facilitator and the institution are doing everything they can to enable success. If feedback–even valid feedback–is provided too late in the course for the student to modify behavior, then feedback is not driving performance and the student is more likely to feel frustration and helplessness. Evaluation comments should be evidence based and not personal. An example of a rating scale developed for use in a small group class is found in Appendix B.

Patients want health care providers who are compassionate and empathic. Fishbein discusses this issue in relation to behavior of physicians (4). He states, "If having compassion implies 'I want to help you,' then empathy suggests that 'I could easily be you.'" The same orientation could apply to faculty and students. Compassion means that faculty are genuinely motivated to assist students. Empathy is identification with how the student feels, and faculty have all had the experience of being students. Boyer described several principles that provided a framework for a community of learning (5). Included in these is "an open community, where freedom of expression is uncompromisingly protected and where civility is powerfully affirmed." Freedom of expression does not mean perpetuating a culture of incivility. Students– and faculty–may require explicit discussion of how to express ideas and dissent without being uncivil. Some have termed this "disagreeing without being disagreeable." Heinemann described the "language of disagreement" as being mostly "respectful listening" (6).

Having stated the above, incivilities may occur and must be addressed directly. As Dr. Berger has discussed, incivilities should not simply be ignored. In small group classes, self-and peer evaluation can be helpful. See Appendix C for characteristics of constructive feedback that students can use in organizing self-assessment and peer assessment comments. This can be delicate, too, especially if done in the public forum of the group. Evidence-based feedback to peers, provided to the facilitator electronically and then anonymously in writing to each student, is one approach. Faculty members should not respond in kind to uncivil acts toward them by students by becoming angry and engaging in arguments. Calm and reasoned discussions with students are the most helpful means of diffusing the incivility. When incivility is followed by incivility, neither party reflects effectively on the behavior that led to the incident. Moreover, when a faculty member responds to the uncivil behavior of a student with additional uncivil behavior, the student is likely to tell his peers about the faculty member's actions. For serious and flagrant offenses such as physical threats or altercations, policies are needed such as honor councils or structured processes to remove the offender, if necessary.

SUMMARY

Incidents of incivility can occur in any setting, including in small group classes. Certain incivilities are less likely to occur in small groups, but the stress of increased scrutiny, demands of preparedness and participation, and alternative methods of assessment may increase the risk of other types of incivilities. Incivilities in whatever form harm the milieu of the class, cause students and faculty to feel uncomfortable or even vulnerable and unsafe, and harm learning. Prosocial behaviors by faculty members, explicit criteria in course syllabi, and frequent evidence-based feedback are keys to preventing and managing incivilities in small group classes.

REFERENCES

1. Organ CH. On the nature of incivility. *Arch Surg.* 2000; 135:395.

2. Lashley FR, de Meneses M. Student civility in nursing programs: A national survey. *J Prof Nurs.* 2001; 17(2):81-6.

3. Berger B. Incivility. *J Pharm Educ.* 2000; 64:445-50.

4. Fishbein RH. Scholarship, humanism, and the young physician. *Acad Med.* 1999; 74:646-51.

5. Boyer EL. In search of community. Paper presented at the American Council on Education, 1990.

6. Heinemann RL. Addressing campus-wide communication incivility in the basic course: A case study. Paper presented at the Annual Meeting of the Speech Communication Association, 1996.

APPENDIX A. Topics for Small Group Class Orientation.

Detailed review of the course syllabus

Philosophical and theoretical basis for small group, student-centered learning

Review of roles and responsibilities of the facilitator and the student

Review of the group routine

Efficient and appropriate use of technology

Review of literature search strategies

Student-initiated resource sessions with faculty experts to supplement the small group

Thorough library orientation

Professional attire policy

Statement on standards of behavior, civility, and respect for differing points of view

APPENDIX B

	Facilitator:
University of Mississippi **School of Pharmacy** **Department of Pharmacy Practice** **Pharmaceutical Care I - IV: Group** **(PRCT 557, 560, 563, 569)** **Facilitator Evaluation of Student Performance**	Student: Date: Class Graduating In: Pharmaceutical Care : Group

KNOWLEDGE: (22%) SCORE: / 35=	%	**WEIGHTED** **TOTAL** **SCORE** **%**
CLINICAL REASONING: (22%) SCORE: / 55=	%	
SELF-DIRECTED LEARNING: (22%) SCORE : / 25 =	%	**FINAL** **ADJUSTED** **SCORE** **%**
INTERPERSONAL AND GROUP SKILLS: (34%) SCORE: / 45=	%	

KNOWLEDGE *Elements of Knowledge Acquisition*	*Score: %*

Given this level of education and training, the student can, when encountering an unfamiliar problem, build, organize, and articulate basic and clinical science knowledge and concepts that can explain the problem and that can be employed to resolve the problem.

1.   The student possesses breadth of knowledge that is integrated from multiple academic disciplines reflected in the course (physiology, pathology, pharmacotherapy, pharmacokinetics, drug literature evaluation).

    5   Discusses knowledge from all disciplines with excellent balance.
    4   Discusses knowledge from all disciplines with good balance but could improve with increased emphasis on certain areas
    3   Discusses knowledge from all disciplines with fair balance, but needs to improve by increased emphasis on certain areas
    2   Discusses knowledge from most disciplines and infrequently discusses knowledge from one or two disciplines.
    1   Most or all discussion is in one or two disciplines; infrequently discusses most areas.

2.   The student possesses knowledge in depth on a variety of topics.

    Discusses information at the level of the basic science mechanism; e.g., at the tissue, cellular or receptor level.

    5   During every group session (3 of 3 weekly sessions).
    4   During most group sessions (2 of 3 weekly sessions).
    3   During some group sessions; at least in every patient case.
    2   During some group sessions; but not in every case.
    1   Does not discuss basic mechanisms.

Elements of Knowledge Acquisition (continued)

3. Able to contrast properties within drug classes following self-directed learning on the drug class.

   5   During every applicable group session.
   4   During most applicable group sessions.
   3   During some applicable group sessions; at least in every patient case.
   2   During some applicable group sessions; but not in every case.
   1   Rarely.

4. Able to discuss knowledge in depth without reading from prepared notes.

   5   During every group session.
   4   During most group sessions.
   3   During some group sessions; at least in every patient case.
   2   During some group sessions; but not in every case.
   1   Rarely.

5. When asked by facilitator, student is able to discuss *all* learning issues identified by the group, not just those that they volunteered to research.

   5   During every group session.
   4   During most group sessions.
   3   During some group sessions; at least in every patient case.
   2   During some group sessions; but not in every case.
   1   Rarely.

6. Knowledge is structured for application to patient problems; i.e., the student does not merely recall information, but can discuss potential significance.

   Knowledge is discussed within the context of the patient problem.

   5   During every group session.
   4   During most group sessions.
   3   During some group sessions; at least in every patient case.
   2   During some group sessions; but not in every case.
   1   Rarely.

7. Knowledge is applied to alternate scenarios that may be presented by the group, such as patients of differing age, ethnic groups, comorbid disease states, pregnancy, etc.

   5   During every applicable group session.
   4   During most applicable group sessions.
   3   During some applicable group sessions; at least in every patient case.
   2   During some applicable group sessions; but not in every case.
   1   Rarely.

APPENDIX B (continued)

CLINICAL REASONING
Steps in the Clinical Reasoning Process   *Score: %*

When presented with a patient problem, the student will demonstrate (orally and/or in writing) clinical reasoning skills in the investigation and resolution of the problem.

1. The student **generates hypotheses** to explain the problem and solutions.

   5   Always generates multiple hypotheses.
   4   Usually generates multiple hypotheses.
   3   Offers at least one hypothesis in nearly all group sessions.
   2   Occasionally offers at least one hypothesis.
   1   Rarely offers hypotheses.

2. Hypotheses are stated in terms of basic mechanisms to explain the problem.

   5 Always   4 Very frequently   3 Usually   2 Occasionally   1 Rarely

3. Identifies evidence or reasoning used in hypothesis formation.

   5 Always   4 Very frequently   3 Usually   2 Occasionally   1 Rarely

4. When applicable, additional data are identified that are needed to discriminate among hypotheses.

   5 Always   4 Very frequently   3 Usually   2 Occasionally   1 Rarely

5. The student will **design an initial recommended treatment plan** to correct the mechanism chosen as responsible for the problem or to alleviate the impact of the problem.

   The plan is logical and the basis for choice of specific agents is included.

   5 Always   4 Not Included Once*   3 Consistently   2 Occasionally   1 Rarely

6. The plan includes a complete dosage regimen design.

   5 Always   4 Not Included Once*   3 Consistently   2 Occasionally   1 Rarely

7. The plan includes patient specific monitoring parameters for therapeutic outcome.

   5 Always   4 Not Included Once*   3 Consistently   2 Occasionally   1 Rarely

8. The plan includes patient specific monitoring parameters for adverse effects.

   5 Always   4 Not Included Once*   3 Consistently   2 Occasionally   1 Rarely

9. The plan includes patient-specific education.

   5 Always   4 Not Included Once*   3 Consistently   2 Occasionally   1 Rarely

10. The plan includes alternate therapy in case of nonresponse to the primary choice. Rationale, dosage, adverse effects and patient education are included.

    5 Always   4 Not Included Once*   3 Consistently   2 Occasionally   1 Rarely

11. The plan is concise and well organized.

    5 Always   4 Except Once*   3 Consistently   2 Occasionally   1 Rarely

* Student always meets criteria after being counseled once

Clinical Reasoning (continued)

SELF-DIRECTED LEARNING
Elements of Self-Directed Learning
Score: %

1. The student **accesses contemporary information**, utilizing an appropriate balance of tertiary and primary literature.

   5 Always; excellent balance between different sources.
   4 Often uses primary literature to complement tertiary sources.
   3 Occasionally uses primary literature to complement tertiary sources.
   2 Infrequently uses primary literature to complement tertiary sources.
   1 Rarely uses primary literature.

2. The student knowledgeably critiques the merits and limitations of primary literature articles brought in during group

   5 Always   4 Usually   3 Occasionally   2 Infrequently   1 Rarely

3. The student knowledgeably critiques the merits and limitations of articles discussed during journal club

   5 Always   4 Usually   3 Occasionally   2 Infrequently   1 Rarely

4. The student properly references all information they present in their work (learning issues, treatment plans, etc.)

   5 Always   4 Usually   3 Occasionally   2 Infrequently   1 Rarely

5. In their learning issues and treatment plans, the student restates information in their own words rather than merely copying information from another source

   5 Always   4 Usually   3 Occasionally   2 Infrequently   1 Rarely.

APPENDIX B (continued)

INTERPERSONAL AND GROUP SKILLS
Elements of Interpersonal and Group Skills   *Score: %*

1. The student **attends every group meeting**. Planned absences should be handled professionally by notifying the facilitator in advance of class. Absences should be for appropriate reasons, not generally for nonprofessional or leisure purposes.

    5   Attends every group meeting.
    4   One excused absence; no unexcused absences.
    3   Two excused absences; no unexcused absences.
    2   More than two excused absences; no unexcused absences.
    1   One unexcused absence.

2. The student is **prepared to begin the group meeting at the scheduled time**.

    5   Attends every group meeting.
    4   Late one time, but called notified facilitator in advance
    3   Arrived late once without notifying facilitator in advance
    2   Late twice, but notified facilitator in advance
    1   Arrived late more than twice, whether or not facilitator was notified

3. The student **actively participates and contributes** to group discussions (provides ideas, uses examples, shares insights).

    5   Consistently initiates and leads discussions.
    4   Participates in all group discussions; occasionally initiates and leads discussions.
    3   Participates in all group discussions.
    2   Tends to be too active (too dominant) or not active enough (too passive).
    1   Frequently is too active (too dominant) or not active enough (too passive).

4. Demonstrates **appropriate interpersonal behavior**; e.g., is not stubborn or defensive about personal opinion, listens actively (avoids sidebar conversations), challenges others in a positive manner when holding a differing opinion.

    5 Always   4 Very frequently   3 Usually   2 Occasionally   1 Rarely

5. The student **augments personal and group learning through the use of visual aids**, diagramming or charting at the board (independent of board scribe responsibility), demonstration of medical devices, etc.

    5 Consistently   4 Frequently   3 Occasionally   2 Rarely   1 Never

6. The student **provides useful self and peer evaluation comments** to reinforce and improve group and individual performance (gives and receives constructive feedback). Specific examples are cited to support comments.

    5   Provides both complimentary and constructive feedback for each student; cites specific evidence for all comments.
    4   Provides both complimentary and constructive feedback for each student; usually cites specific evidence for all comments.
    3   Provides comments about all peers; usually includes constructive suggestions as well complimentary feedback; usually cites specific evidence for all comments.
    2   Makes only nonspecific or complimentary remarks about peers.
    1   Fails to submit peer evaluation comments on one occasion.

7. The student **demonstrates a caring attitude** toward patients being discussed. Willingness to provide assistance and care to patients should be evident, even when specific disease topics, lifestyle behaviors or cultural factors may be regarded as unusual or unpleasant.

    5   Always.
    3   Consistently; does not indicate unwillingness to care for patients after counseling on a single incident.
    1   Repeated refuses to care for patients despite counseling.

Interpersonal and Group Skills (continued)

---

8. The student **demonstrates a respectful and professional demeanor** in interactions with peers and faculty members.

   5   Always.
   3   Consistently; does not repeat disrespectful or unprofessional behavior after counseling on a single incident.
   2   Repeats disrespectful or unprofessional behavior.
   1   Often disrespectful or unprofessional.

9. The student should be **neatly and professionally attired and groomed**.

   5   Always.
   4   Maintains attire and grooming after counseling on one incident.
   3   Maintains attire and grooming after counseling on two incidents.
   1   More than one incident on failure to maintain professional attire or grooming.

APPENDIX C. Characteristics of Constructive Feedback (considerations in participating in assessment of performance in group).

1. Think about why you are giving feedback. The most important goal of assessment is to improve and optimize performance, not merely to measure it. To accomplish this goal, feedback must be early and frequent.

2. Assessment must be self-reflective as well as provided to others. Effective practice of pharmacy requires that we assess ourselves to improve provision of care.

3. Comments to others should be based on specific observed behavior that is fully described rather than generalizations. As such, assessment is evidence based and depersonalized.

4. Comments aimed to improve performance should be framed in terms that allow for improvement. Specific suggestions for change are helpful. Pointing out problems over which the recipient has no control only causes frustration.

5. Prioritize feedback and consider the recipient's ability to absorb and act. The most important comments should have the greatest emphasis. Do not avoid addressing important concerns by mentioning only minor issues.

6. Feedback should be individually referenced, not comparative. Refrain from comparing others to the group or class.

7. Use the "sandwich" technique. Place negative feedback between two pieces of positive feedback. Start with at least one piece of positive feedback, follow up with the negative feedback, then conclude with additional positive feedback.

Experiential Learning: Transitioning Students from Civility to Professionalism

Diane E. Beck
Janelle L. Krueger
Debbie C. Byrd

INTRODUCTION

The experiential component of a pharmacy curriculum includes both introductory and advanced practice experiences that occur as a continuum across the curriculum. The introductory pharmacy practice experiences (IPPEs) are expected to begin early in the curriculum and allow the student to progressively develop the ability to provide pharmaceutical care. Advanced pharmacy practice experiences (APPEs) are capstone experiences that provide students with in-depth practice in a

Diane E. Beck, Pharm.D., is Director of Experiential Learning and Professor, Harrison School of Pharmacy, Auburn University, 217 Walker Pharmacy Building, Auburn, AL 36849 (E-mail: beckdia@auburn.edu). Janelle L. Krueger, M.S., is Coordinator of the Introductory Pharmacy Practice Experience Program and Assistant Clinical Professor, Harrison School of Pharmacy, Auburn University (E-mail: Kruegjl@auburn.edu). Debbie C. Byrd, Pharm.D., is Associate Professor, Harrison School of Pharmacy, Auburn University, and Clinical Associate Professor of Family Medicine, College of Community Health Sciences, University of Alabama, Tuscaloosa, AL 35401 (E-mail: byrddeb@auburn.edu).

[Haworth co-indexing entry note]: "Experiential Learning: Transitioning Students from Civility to Professionalism." Beck, Diane E., Janelle L. Krueger, and Debbie C. Byrd. Co-published simultaneously in *Journal of Pharmacy Teaching* (Pharmaceutical Products Press, an imprint of The Haworth Press, Inc.) Vol. 9, No. 3, 2002, pp. 37-55; and: *Promoting Civility in Pharmacy Education* (ed: Bruce A. Berger) Pharmaceutical Products Press, an imprint of The Haworth Press, Inc., 2003, pp. 37-55. Single or multiple copies of this article are available for a fee from The Haworth Document Delivery Service [1-800-HAWORTH, 9:00 a.m. - 5:00 p.m. (EST). E-mail address: docdelivery@haworthpress.com].

http://www.haworthpress.com/store/product.asp?sku=J060
© 2003 by The Haworth Press, Inc. All rights reserved.

10.1300/J060v09n03_04

variety of patient care settings. These final experiences allow students to "develop, in a graded fashion, the level of confidence and responsibility needed for independent and collaborative practice" (1).

Because these experiences occur in actual practice settings, students encounter situations where they are expected to demonstrate civil and professional behaviors. The goals of this paper are to:

1. Characterize the dimensions of civility most relevant to experiential practice settings and identify the types of incivility most commonly seen in experiential learning
2. Recommend strategies for responding to incivilities at both the programmatic and individual instructor levels
3. Recommend implementation of a code of professional conduct that can guide students in developing and demonstrating civility and other aspects of professional behavior as they progress from IPPEs through the APPE sequence.

FRAME OF REFERENCE

The recommendations provided in this paper are based on a review of the social sciences and health professions literature. The example cases are based on our experiences in conducting a longitudinal introductory practice experience and a ten-month advanced practice experience at Auburn University. One of the ten ability-based outcomes for the Auburn Pharm.D. program is "Professional Ethics and Identity," and students are expected to show developmental growth in achieving this outcome as they progress across both the IPPE and APPE experiences. This outcome includes criteria related to civility.

Our IPPE is unique in that students are assigned to a pharmacy team during orientation to pharmacy school. Throughout the first three years, students visit a patient on a weekly basis and report their progress to faculty mentors during weekly team meetings. One of the primary reasons for this continuous experience model is to promote the professional socialization of our pharmacy students (2).

Our advanced practice experience sequence is designed to document the final growth and achievement of the Pharm.D. program's ten ability-based outcomes by students. Because our students have had three years of patient care and team responsibilities by the time they begin their APPEs, they are accountable for demonstrating a higher level of ability for the "Professional Ethics and Identity" outcome as compared to eight other program outcomes when they begin the APPE sequence. Unsatisfactory achievement in this single outcome can result in failure of a rotation even though the student has excelled in all other outcome areas. The following literature review and discussion will provide the reader a means for understanding the rationale for this continuous experiential learning model.

LITERATURE REVIEW

Civility and Today's Students

Civility is often interpreted as politeness. However, Carter has proposed that we define civility in broader terms (3). He specifically points out that living in society is like living in a household. Carter notes that in a household, moral people maintain relationships with other people according to standards of behavior and that, at times, these standards may limit an individual's freedom. A civil person follows standards of behavior even though the person may not agree with or like other individuals in the household (or society). This analogy illustrates that, in the past, rules of civility were instilled during childhood. Carter and others have pointed out that, in addition to a decreased emphasis in teaching children rules of civility, other factors, such as the introduction of technology, have contributed to an overall decline in civility in our society (3, 4).

Faculty need to be cognizant that many of the young adults entering pharmacy school, and thus IPPEs, have not been inculcated with standards of behavior prior to starting pharmacy school (3). Such students may not be prepared to "make sacrifices for the sake of living together in a community where their patients exist" and work in the "health professions household" (3). Experiential programs, therefore, need to clearly communicate expected standards of behavior when IPPEs begin, explain how these standards relate to professionalism, and hold students accountable for meeting a code of professional conduct throughout all practice experiences.

Incivility in the Practice Setting

In the practice setting, students may succumb to incivility as they interact with faculty, other health professionals/teams, and patients. However, the occurrence of incivilities is a two-way path; although we most often think of students demonstrating incivility, they may also be recipients as they communicate with faculty, other health professionals/teams, and patients.

Students often will not discuss or disclose incidents of incivility involving faculty members because they fear that the faculty member will retaliate or that the administration will not believe them. Medical educators have documented that when medical students are subjected to abuse and exposed to unprofessional behaviors, the conflict may cause them to abandon the desired attitudes and behaviors they were initially taught to exhibit (5). Hundert has recommended that programs offer students opportunities, without faculty present, to discuss incidents that contradict the ideal attitudes and behaviors they have been taught (6).

Tiberius and Flak point out that in one-on-one teaching and learning situations, such as practice experiences, extreme forms of incivility like those occurring in the large classroom setting are rarely overtly displayed (7). For example, the loud talking, sarcastic remarks, or emotional outbursts that have been reported in the large classroom setting rarely occur in small group situations (8). Tiberius and Flak have noted that when students interact with a faculty member in a one-on-one or small group encounter, they are more likely to exhibit withdrawal and uncooperativeness or to hold out and express inappropriate negativity in a written end-of-course evaluation (7). Pharmacy students are, therefore, more likely to exhibit passive-aggressive behaviors in one-on-one or small group interactions with experiential faculty members.

The primary types of incivility most likely to occur in the experiential practice setting are listed in Table 1. These examples of incivility are categorized according to four dimensions of civility that are common themes in the current literature describing how to live a civil life in society (3). In the section below, we briefly define each dimension, provide examples of how faculty members and students may role model civility and/or exhibit incivility, and give suggestions for promoting civility or addressing incivility.

Tolerance. Given the number of people who enter the practice setting (e.g., patients, faculty, other health professionals, staff, and students), it should be anticipated that a variety of cultures will be represented. Each culture has a set of beliefs, values, and lifestyles that shapes how members of that culture perceive and experience life. Our pharmacy graduates must be culturally competent and effectively relate to patients, colleagues, and staff who are different from them. Experiential rotations take place in a real-world setting where students must interact with

TABLE 1. Civility and Incivility in the Practice Setting.

Dimensions of Civility	Examples of Incivilities
Tolerance	**Faculty Member** • Making derogatory comments to other students or faculty members about an upcoming student who has a different lifestyle or value (e.g., gender, race, sexual preference, religious preference, socioeconomic class) **Student** • Making derogatory comments to other team members or peers about a patient's lifestyle or value (e.g., gender, race, sexual preference, religious preference, socioeconomic class) • Intolerance for ambiguity and anxiety[30]
Respect	**Faculty Member** • Making derogatory comments to other students or faculty members about the role and value of those in another discipline (e.g., basic sciences, medical profession, nursing profession) • Not respecting the student as a learner even though he or she has made a sincere effort to learn • When providing feedback about performance, using derogatory or nasty language • Public belittlement and humiliation in the presence of others in the clinical setting • Not treating students as colleagues **Student** • Not following assignments or disobeying orders given by pharmacists, pharmacy residents, or fellows when the faculty member has designated the individual as a colleague faculty member during the rotation • Nonparticipative and uncooperative behavior in teaching sessions held by a pharmacist, pharmacy resident, or fellow (The experiential faculty member has designated the individual to be the instructor for the teaching session.) • Refusing to follow orders and accept constructive criticism from a faculty member who is young or inexperienced • Not seeking patient desires for how to be addressed (first name or Mr./Ms.) • Not using appropriate titles in the practice area (e.g., calling faculty members by first name and not using "Dr." or "Ms.") • Lack of courtesy
Conduct	**Faculty Member** • Telling the students to meet at a given time but showing up late or not showing up at all • Using foul language or referring to the student in a derogatory manner during a learning session

TABLE 1 (continued)

Dimensions of Civility	Examples of Incivilities
Conduct (continued)	**Student** • Poor grooming and/or not following the dress code established by the practice site • Using foul language in a patient care area • Sitting around and joking with peer students in a patient care area • Not following guidelines established by the faculty member or medical team (e.g., arriving late to the practice site or rounds, not wearing proper identification) • Not being an active participant on the medical team • Not being polite with patients and staff (e.g., not using please and thank you when talking or giving directions) • Complaining about a program policy to the experiential faculty member such that it interferes with patient care or disrupts the site
Diplomacy	**Faculty Member** • Reacting negatively when a student respectfully disagrees with a faculty member's viewpoint • Not giving a student the opportunity to express his or her viewpoint and/or not listening to the student's perspective • Assuming the faculty member is always right and the student is always wrong **Student** • Constantly argumentative about rotation activities and requirements • Inappropriate reactions to constructive feedback • Not informing the faculty member of concerns about the teaching approach or learning experience during the rotation and instead writing offensive and angry comments on the Teaching and Site Evaluation Form • Not resolving conflicts in a manner that respects the dignity of all people involved[24] • Not listening to others

people of various cultures, providing students with the best environment for learning and demonstrating cultural competency.

Although most individuals know better than to make derogatory statements about a person's gender, race, sexual preference, religious preference, or socioeconomic class in the practice setting with others present, incidents involving both medical residents and students have been reported in the medical education literature (9). Such cases have not been documented in the pharmacy education literature, but we should expect them to occur with pharmacy students, given the similarity of medical rotations and pharmacy rotations.

Experiential faculty members should be mindful that cultural insensitivities probably occur more often than we realize and may go unrecognized by a faculty member who has not been trained in cultural competency and is not sensitive to implicit messages that can sometimes be conveyed in daily life. Medical educators have cautioned that students can learn attitudes and values from incidents of incivility committed unwittingly by faculty members and that these incidents are often counter to what students are supposed to learn according to the formal curriculum. Medical educators have cautioned about the effects of this "hidden or informal curriculum" (5). For example, Finucane et al. have reported incidents where case reports included descriptions that promoted racial stereotyping (10). Experiential faculty should also carefully evaluate stories and jokes that are shared among the team during a rotation experience and assess whether they convey a cultural bias. These situations accentuate the importance of maintaining careful vigilance for cultural bias, which may be very subtle but still weaken the formal curriculum.

Uncivil statements may be made by peer students and other health professionals when the preceptor is not present, and these undermine the attitudes and behaviors that are taught in the formal curriculum. For example, as students travel together to practice sites and share their rotation experiences, they may make statements that are culturally inappropriate. Cultural sensitivity training programs can enable peer students to detect such inappropriate behaviors and help them address their peer's behaviors in an appropriate manner (11).

Respect. The American Board of Internal Medicine has noted that "respect for others (patients and their families, other physicians, and professional colleagues such as nurses, medical students, residents, and subspecialty fellows) is the essence of humanism" (12). The board further notes that humanism is a central characteristic of professionalism. Because pharmaceutical care calls for pharmacists to be patient "caring," pharmacy education needs to place greater emphasis on helping pharmacy students develop humanistic skills.

Reiser has pointed out that the student-teacher relationship molds the quality of the student-patient relationship and, eventually, the practitioner-patient relationship (13, 14). The Hippocratic Oath, which is the ethical foundation for medicine, emphasizes that the student and teacher should relate as "members of a family." Pharmacy faculty members who demonstrate caring to pharmacy students will better prepare students to provide pharmaceutical care. As noted in Table 1, faculty role model incivility when they make disparaging comments about other pharmacy faculty members, the school administration, or other health professionals in the presence of students.

Students demonstrate incivility when they are disrespectful to the experiential faculty member or a designated instructor such as a pharmacy resident or fellow. Both the literature and our experience confirm that this occurs more frequently with new faculty members who set high standards (sometimes unrealistic for the learner) (15).

We have also encountered pharmacy students who show respect to the experiential faculty member but are disrespectful to a pharmacy resident or fellow designated by the faculty member to help instruct or supervise the student. Students should be told during orientation that residents and fellows must be given the same level of respect given to the experiential faculty member. Furthermore, if the residents and fellows are involved in providing instruction or supervision, they should provide input into the assessment of student professionalism.

Conduct. Carter has emphasized that living with others requires that we conform to an established set of behaviors (3). In the practice setting, these behaviors include using of appropriate language, wearing professional attire, grooming properly, and participating actively in team rounds rather than being a passive observer or displaying inappropriate behaviors such as joking or talking with peers about topics that are not patient related.

It is important for the experiential faculty member to communicate standards of behavior that are the culture of the team at the beginning of the rotation and also to role model the expected behaviors. For example, during orientation, students should be advised that they are expected to be on time and to have all patient data updated before rounds begin. They should be instructed to be attentive on rounds, and if two pharmacy students are on the same team, they should not converse with each other while another team member is talking. Students need to be reminded that cell phones are prohibited in hospitals and that it is absolutely unacceptable to have their cell phones on.

With pharmacy education's greater emphasis on ambulatory rotations, students spend less time participating in formal inpatient rounds and therefore have only a limited time to learn how to be an integral member of an inpatient team. Students need specific orientation to the standards of behavior expected during team rounds. Faculty members should also round with the team so they can serve as role models, observe the students' behaviors, and provide feedback about this performance.

Diplomacy. Civility does not imply that an individual should always conform and agree with others. Carter emphasizes that criticism is appropriate and valuable as long as it is civil (3). Faculty members can role model this by encouraging students to express their viewpoints and by promoting civil debate of controversial topics. Diplomacy is also role modeled when the faculty member constructively criticizes a student's performance. For example, when providing feedback about performance, the faculty member should describe the inappropriate behaviors (e.g., your plans for solving medication-related problems are often incorrect) rather than labeling the student by using a demeaning term such as "dumb" or "lazy." Furthermore, the student should not be belittled in the presence of others, especially patients, when a task is performed inappropriately.

Students should be encouraged to share their concerns about the quality of the learning experience during the rotation rather than letting emotions build up and writing offensive comments about the faculty member on the Student Evaluation of Teaching form. Students tend to resist providing negative feedback about the instruction during a rotation for fear of retaliation or negative impact on their final rotation grade. The faculty member can minimize this by establishing a teacher-student bond at the beginning of the rotation and encouraging constructive feedback for the purpose of maximizing the student's learning. This point is discussed in more detail below.

STRATEGIES FOR PREVENTING AND MANAGING INCIVILITY

As described by Tiberius and Flak, it has been our experience that students fear faculty retaliation and are hesitant to openly express even appropriate emotions (7). Recent incidents that have occurred with graduate students, another form of one-on-one interaction, suggest that these relationships have the potential for culminating in explosive and catastrophic situations (4). Experiential faculty and administrators need skills for addressing even the most subtle occurrences of incivility. The following discussion outlines strategies that can be implemented at the programmatic and individual faculty levels to prevent and manage incidents of incivility.

Programmatic Strategies

As noted in the ACPE accreditation standards, the experiential component of the curriculum should occur as a continuum across the curriculum and allow students to progressively develop the ability to provide pharmaceutical care (16). Most pharmacy schools have adopted a set of learning outcomes, and one of these outcomes should communicate that ethics and professionalism must be demonstrated by the successful graduate. Because practice experiences are intended to be a continuum across the curriculum, they provide the most appropriate venue for enabling students to grow and to demonstrate civility and professionalism in the practice setting. The formal experiential curriculum should provide students with opportunities to demonstrate achievement of civility, other virtues, and professionalism in a graded fashion over time.

As described below, pharmacy students must learn that virtues are the foundation for professionalism. Students need more than just knowledge about virtues and other aspects of professionalism. We must help them make use of virtues and professionalism a daily habit as they progress across the entire experiential sequence. This can be promoted by allowing students to reflect on their patient care experiences and to discuss the ethical and professional dilemmas they have encountered.

Virtues such as civility have been cited by various health professions faculty members as important foundations for understanding ethics and demonstrating professionalism (17-20). Pellegrino and Thomasma state that "virtue makes us function well as humans to achieve our purposes" (17). A virtue defines human excellence, and adherence to virtues makes good humans. Other virtues that are particularly germane to the health professions include fidelity to trust, compassion, phronesis (prudence), justice, fortitude, temperance, integrity, and altruism (17).

We recommend that pharmacy students be introduced to virtues by the time they begin their first IPPE. Specifically, students should be taught about the virtues that are essential for excellent pharmacy practice, how these enable one to develop a sense of morals or ethics, and that morals are a prelude for effectively interacting with others (3). As noted by Anderson, it is probably unrealistic to expect students to begin a professional program such as medical school or pharmacy school with an understanding of all of the virtues that relate to their career (18). Students need to be nurtured as they learn about virtues and need to be provided with opportunities to make use of virtues a habit. All experiential faculty members need to role model these virtues and to encourage students to apply them each day and to reflect on their experiences (19). For example, during orientation to the first IPPE, students should be provided guidance in how to interact with others in a civil manner and told that civility is the foundation for professionalism.

As pharmacy students continue in their early practice experiences, they should be held accountable for behaving in a civil manner. Students should then be held accountable for demonstrating professional behaviors, including civility, during their APPE sequence.

Many incidents of incivility can be prevented if a code of professional conduct is established at the programmatic level and clearly communicated when students begin the IPPE sequence. Many programs have policies that mandate attendance, dress, and standards of behavior that in reality relate to civility and professionalism. However, students often view these policies as "course rules" and do not realize that they represent behaviors of professionalism.

Based on several recent incidents, we believe our students may better understand the rationale for our program policies related to attendance, dress, and use of professional language if we incorporate them into a code of professional conduct. To establish such a code, readers are encouraged to review the work of Hammer and the recent Charter of Professionalism that physicians developed during the Medical Professionalism Project (12, 21-23). Pharmacy schools are also encouraged to consider a system for longitudinally detecting professionalism problems as students progress across the curriculum (24). Furthermore, there should be severe consequences if this code is breeched so that students get the message that attitudes and values are as important as knowledge and skills in pharmacy practice. For example, as noted in the introduction, Auburn students must achieve a higher level of performance on the ratings related to the Professional Ethics and Identity outcome because they participate in a longitudinal practice experience that enables their growth as professionals. If students fail to achieve a minimum standard of performance on the Professional Ethics and Identity outcome at the end of an APPE rotation, they fail the rotation even though they have excelled in all other outcome areas. This performance criterion sends students the message that pharmacy practice involves more than just knowledge and skills; professional attitudes and values are essential in providing pharmaceutical care.

In addition to individual faculty member ratings that assess performance related to the Professional Ethics and Identity outcome at the end of each rotation, the Auburn Experiential Program faculty meets to review the progress of each student at the midpoint and end of the year. These discussions enable the faculty to assess the strengths and weaknesses of each individual student and recommend strategies for improvement. By having faculty members share their insights about a student's performance with other faculty members, we have been able to detect problems faculty members were hesitant to document in writing. These sessions have also enabled the faculty to confirm whether a student's weakness or performance problem has been consistent across rotations and whether improvement and growth have occurred. These faculty evaluation sessions review the progress of students in accomplishing all ten of the program outcomes. They also allow the faculty to collaboratively develop a plan for helping the student improve. The information is then provided to students for use in personal improvement.

Hemmer et al. have shown that faculty evaluation sessions such as this are more likely to detect medical student behavior and professionalism problems than standard checklists (e.g., ratings) or written comments (25). These researchers also found that professionalism deficiencies were more likely to be detected in the inpatient setting than in the ambulatory care setting. Because of the increased emphasis on ambulatory care, students are spending less time in the formal inpatient setting and pharmacy educators should be aware that this may make detection of professionalism problems more difficult.

The faculty evaluation sessions also enable faculty development because the more inexperienced faculty members gain insight from those more experienced about how they observe students, the level of performance they expect, and their interpretation of the findings. These faculty reviews of student progress have been successful, and some faculty members have encouraged us to perform reviews more frequently than twice a year.

Some readers may be questioning the legal ramifications of failing or even expelling a student based on performance in the areas of civility and professionalism and whether it is appropriate to share student performance data with other experiential faculty members during faculty review sessions. In both situations, the courts have upheld the faculty member's activities and decisions (26-28).

Routine site visits and meetings with students provide opportunities for the program director to assess the frequency of incidents where faculty members are exhibiting incivility in their daily practice or treating students in an uncivil manner. The director can also determine whether patients have been uncivil to students. Each of these situations has been detected in our program as a result of routine site visits. Fortunately, during a 15-year period, only one incident has occurred where the experiential faculty member was exhibiting incivility in daily practice. This individual and site were subsequently dropped from the program. Although there have been some incidents where an experiential faculty member demonstrated incivility related to tolerance and conduct, incidents related to treating the student with respect or humanism and using diplomacy when interacting with the student have been more frequent.

Students do encounter situations where patients are uncivil because they are frustrated with the pharmacy operations (e.g., perceived slow service). We have also encountered situations where patients insisted on talking to a "male pharmacist" because the student was a female. In one incident, it was very traumatic for the female student because it had occurred multiple times in a single rotation. The program director provided a reflective session with the student to help the student understand that some patients are accustomed to interacting with a male pharmacist or may feel more comfortable talking about health care issues with a pharmacist of the same gender. During the discussion, it was emphasized that once the student is in daily practice, she will have opportunity to gain the confidence of such patients over time.

Faculty Member Strategies

Experiential faculty members should be prepared to both prevent incivility and manage a situation if it occurs. Tiberius and Flak emphasize that building a strong teacher-learner alliance provides an atmosphere where the faculty member and the student can have an effective relationship, one where they feel comfortable sharing concerns with each other in an open manner (7). The following recommendations for building a strong teacher-learner alliance are supported by their research and expertise.

At the beginning of a rotation, the teacher-learner alliance can be achieved by establishing an atmosphere where both commit to working together to help the student achieve the rotation goals and take a shared responsibility in helping the student learn and improve. Both the student and the faculty member should agree to hold weekly sessions to provide feedback to each other about the student's progress and how learning can be enhanced. The student should be particularly encouraged to share ways that the experiential faculty member can enhance the learning environment. The faculty member can role model humility by emphasizing that he or she is also an imperfect human being and desires feedback so he or she can improve learning during the rotation. Although a faculty member usually has more expertise and may have superior understanding of a topic, the student should be encouraged to express his or her perspectives on a topic or issue. By listening carefully and providing civil feedback, the instructor has an opportunity to correct or clarify misinterpretations that may otherwise go undetected. Students can learn significantly from these new understandings.

The faculty member should also be prepared to intervene and address issues or incidents where incivility is likely to result. Table 2 outlines seven steps recommended by Tiberius and Flak for communicating effectively when issues arise (7).

EXAMPLE STUDENT CASES AND DISCUSSION

The following example student cases highlight some of the issues and recommendations we have discussed in this article and provide further thought on issues related to incivility in the experiential learning setting.

IPPE Student Case

Shortly after being assigned to visit a patient in a nearby community, a female student contacted the experiential program director (JLK) and requested reassignment to another patient in Auburn. The nearby com-

TABLE 2. Steps for Resolving an Experiential Faculty Member-Student Issue and Preventing Incivility [recommendations cited by Tiberius and Flak (7)].

Steps	Description
Step 1	Detect early warning signs and symptoms: (irritability, loss of motivation, insomnia, and headaches)
Step 2	Schedule a mutually agreeable time to meet (allow sufficient time and privacy)
Step 3	Use active listening techniques (e.g., paraphrasing what the student has told you and checking for accuracy)
Step 4	Confirm and validate the student's statement of the problem (Clearly indicate you agree or differ)
Step 5	Express empathy for the student (use verbal and nonverbal techniques)
Step 6	Explain your viewpoint to each other (each should use the pronoun "I" instead of "you")
Step 7	Establish solutions (Initially, both individuals should brainstorm and then narrow down to the best option.)

munity, twenty miles from campus, has a high percentage of both im-
poverished and minority residents. The student expressed concerns
about having to drive a distance to visit the patient and further shared
that visiting patients in that community did not seem "safe" to her (even
though she had never visited the community). The coordinator assured
the student that the patient did not live in a "dangerous" area and detected that the problem more likely related to student misperceptions
about the patient's culture and neighborhood. She encouraged the student to talk with her individual faculty member (DEB) and express
these concerns.

When the student approached the faculty member about her concerns, the faculty member detected that the student was equating poor
living conditions with danger. The student also shared that she had discussed the assignment with her parents and that they did not want her
going to that community. The faculty member clarified the difference
between "poor" and "dangerous" and then shared her experiences in
visiting the patient and neighborhood. She then arranged for the student
to visit the patient with a senior student who had experience in caring
for the patient. Both students were encouraged to give the patient the
same level of care they would give to their parents, who are from a traditional middle-class background. Following the visit, the faculty member had both students share their experiences and assess the difference
between living in a senior living facility that has poor citizens and walking down a street that is known for violence and therefore, "dangerous."
The student later admitted that her initial perceptions of the community
were formed by the opinions of other students.

Case Commentary

Students often will not express overt intolerance for people of another culture or social status. Instead, they try to avoid the rotation assignment or situation. When students make such requests, faculty should
use open-ended questions and active listening to assess whether the un-
derlying etiology is related to fears or biases about the patient's culture.
This case had the potential for escalating to a point where the student refused to accept the rotation assignment and pulled her parents into the
issue. Through active listening and giving both students an opportunity
to reflect on their experiences, both the program coordinator and the individual faculty member provided an environment that allowed the student to realize her preconceived biases and to learn about a patient from
another culture who was poor, but living in a safe neighborhood.

The student's statement that her initial opinions were based on the opinions of other students suggests the presence of a "hidden curriculum." Because similar incidents have occurred with prior students, the program director recommended that the school train faculty to detect and address cultural issues and implement a series of seminars to enhance the culture competency of students.

APPE Student Case

Early in the rotation sequence, a student was reported to have missed some rotation days and to be habitually tardy during several rotations. During an internal medicine rotation, she was late for rounds several times and it was disruptive to the team. Because the problem had not improved during the rotation, the faculty member contacted the program director for assistance. The experiential director (DEB) met with the student to discuss the problem, and the student revealed that she had been dealing with some personal family problems since the APPE rotations had started. She further shared that during the last several months she had found herself having difficulty getting out of bed in the morning and feeling depressed. She revealed that, through self-referral, she had sought psychiatric treatment for depression and had been taking an antidepressant for about one month. Although her depression could account for her absences and tardiness in earlier rotations, she acknowledged that she had always had difficulty being on time.

Knowing that her upcoming experiential faculty member (DCB) had heard through the "grapevine" that the student had attendance problems, the program director encouraged her to share her situation with the upcoming preceptor so that the upcoming experiential faculty member could assist her in overcoming the problem. Prior to meeting with the student, this experiential faculty member (DCB) developed a clearly written attendance policy that was added to her syllabus, and she began requiring that students sign an affidavit indicating that they understood the policy. The student met with the faculty member prior to the rotation, and they openly discussed the student's past problems and the expectation of arriving to rounds on time and ready to make patient care recommendations. The experiential faculty member conveyed the standards of behavior that the medical team expected and emphasized that arriving late was disruptive to the team. During the rotation, the experiential faculty member had to address one tardiness issue. She was very firm about the issue and pointed out that one more incident would result in failure of the rotation. The student did successfully complete the rotation and after graduation contacted the experiential faculty member and thanked her for helping her overcome habitual tardiness.

Case Commentary

When a student does not follow the established standards of behavior, the faculty member needs to openly discuss the situation with the student and assess the possible etiologies. Although tardiness may seem to be a minor incivility, it continued in spite of directions from earlier faculty members to be on time for rounds. The etiology of the student's attendance problem was most likely a combination of both her depressive illness and a habit she had developed during her early college years of not arriving to class on time.

This student had already sought treatment for her depression, and the faculty were not presented with the challenge of detecting that the incivility was due to a psychiatric problem that needed to be addressed to solve the problem. We have encountered instances where students have exhibited performance problems that called for mandatory psychotherapy. Amada has noted that psychiatric problems are a frequent cause of incivility in college students today (29). However, when such treatment is mandated by the school and the student is not open to it, treatment is unlikely to be successful. Furthermore, Amada notes that this is probably a violation of Section 504 of the Rehabilitation Act of 1973 (29). When readers encounter such a situation, they are encouraged to read the article by Amada and seek assistance from an individual at the university who is familiar with the legal ramifications of any proposed action.

SUMMARY

Incivility during experiential practice rotations usually presents differently from incivility in the large classroom setting. Since incivility and other virtues provide the foundation for professionalism, it is essential that students learn established standards of behavior early in their IPPEs and learn how to live in the "patient care household." They should also be aware of other virtues that serve as the foundation for professionalism and be encouraged to make them daily habits. As Pharm.D. students progress to their APPEs, they will be better prepared to effectively care for patients, interact with others from different cultures, demonstrate respect for others, follow the standards of behavior established by medical teams, and disagree in a diplomatic manner. Experiential programs should evaluate their established policies. If the policies really convey a code of professional conduct, rename the document so that students learn they are following these rules because they are "professionals" and not just students in an educational program with rules and regulations. Finally, as students progress across their APPE sequence, they should be accountable for demonstrating professionalism as outlined in a code of professional conduct that has been adopted by the experiential program.

REFERENCES

1. ACPE. Standards 2000. Chicago: American Council on Pharmaceutical Education; 2000.
2. Beck DE, Thomas SG, Janer AL. Introductory practice experiences: A conceptual framework. *Am J Pharm Educ*. 1996; 60:122-31.
3. Carter SL. Civility. New York: Basic Books; 1998.
4. Morrissette PJ. Reducing incivility in the university/college classroom. *Int Electron J Leadership Learn*. 2001; 5(4). Available at http://www.ucalgary.ca/~iejll/volume5/morrissette.html. Accessed 1 Mar 2001.
5. Hafferty FW, Franks R. The hidden curriculum, ethics teaching, and the structure of medical education. *Acad. Med*. 1998; 69:861-71.
6. Hundert EM. Characteristics of the informal curriculum and trainees' ethical choices. *Acad Med*. 1996; 71:624-33.
7. Tiberius RG, Flak E. Incivility in dyadic teaching and learning. *N Directions Teach Learn*. 1999; 77:3-12.
8. Boice B. Classroom incivilities. *Res Higher Educ*. 1996; 37:453-87.
9. Johnston MAC. Reflections on experiences with socially active students. In: Educating for professionalism: creating a culture of humanism in medical education. Wear D, Bickel J, eds. Iowa City: University of Iowa Press; 2000:95-104.
10. Finucane TE, Carrese JA. Racial bias in presentations of cases. *J Gen Intern Med*. 1990; 5:120-1.
11. Robins LS, Fantone JC, Hermann J, et al. Improving cultural awareness and sensitivity training in medical school. *Acad Med*. 1998; 73(Suppl):S31-S34.
12. American Board of Internal Medicine. Project professionalism. Philadelphia: American Board of Internal Medicine; 2001. Available at: http://www.abim.org. Accessed 28 Feb 2002.
13. Reiser SJ. The ethics of learning and teaching medicine. *Acad Med*. 1994; 69:872-6.
14. Reiser SJ. The moral order of the medical school . . . In: Educating for professionalism: creating a culture of humanism in medical education. Wear D, Bickel J, eds. Iowa City: University of Iowa Press; 2000:3-10.
15. Kuhlenschmidt SL. Promoting internal civility: Understanding our beliefs about teaching and students. *N Directions Teach Learn*. 1999; 77:13-22.

16. ACPE. Accreditation standards and guidelines for the professional program in pharmacy leading to the Doctor of Pharmacy degree adopted June 14, 1997 and implementation procedures. Chicago: American Council on Pharmaceutical Education; 1997.

17. Pellegrino ED, Thomasma DC. The virtues in medical practice. New York: Oxford University Press; 1993.

18. Anderson RE, Obenshain SS. Cheating by students: Findings, reflections, and remedies. *Acad Med.* 1994; 69:323-32.

19. Green MJ, Mitchell G, Stocking CB, et al. Do actions reported by physicians in training conflict with consensus guidelines on ethics? *Arch Intern Med.* 1996; 156: 298-304.

20. Coulehan J, Williams PC. Vanquishing virtue: The impact of medical education. *Acad Med.* 2001; 76:598-605.

21. Hammer DP, Mason HL, Chalmers RK, Popovich NG, Rupp MT. Development and testing of an instrument to assess behavioral professionalism of pharmacy students. *Am J Pharm Educ.* 2000; 64:141-51.

22. Hammer DP. Professional attitudes and behaviors: The "A's and B's" of professionalism. *Am J Pharm Educ.* 2000; 64:455-64.

23. Medical Professionalism Project. Medical professionalism in the new millennium: A physicians' charter. *Ann Intern Med.* 2002; 136:243-6.

24. Papadakis M, Loeser H, Healy K. Early detection and evaluation of professionalism deficiencies in medical students: One school's approach. *Acad Med.* 2001; 76:1100-6.

25. Hemmer PA, Hawkins R, Jackson JL, Pangaro LN. Assessing how well three evaluation methods detect deficiencies in medical students' professionalism in two settings of an internal medicine clerkship. *Acad Med.* 2000; 76:167-73.

26. Irby DM, Milam S. The legal context for evaluating and dismissing medical students and residents. *Acad Med.* 1989; 64:639-43.

27. *Regents of the University of Michigan v. Ewing*, 474 U.S. 214, 106 S.Ct. 507, 88 L.Ed.2d 523 (1985).

28. *Board of Curators of the University of Missouri v. Horowitz*, 435 U.S. 78, 98 S.Ct. 948, 55 L.Ed.2d 124 (1978).

29. Amada G. Coping with the disruptive college student: A practical model. *J Am Coll Health.* 1992; 40:203-15.

30. Epstein ER, Hundert EM. Defining and assessing professional competence. *JAMA* 2002; 287:226-35.

Promoting Civility
in Graduate Student Education

Holly L. Mason

INTRODUCTION

Civil behavior in a graduate program is a key underpinning that predicts overall success for the participants in the program. Both faculty members and students can be on the giving and receiving end of uncivil behavior. Because faculty members typically have more experience and a more fully developed set of behavioral standards, they tend more often to be the recipients of uncivil behavior. However, when uncivil behavior is demonstrated by a faculty member toward a graduate student, there is more potential for harm to the recipient. Bruce Berger, in his introductory article, refers to incivility as "speech or action that is disrespectful or rude" (1). Although this definition is adequate for the purposes of this article, it should be noted that incivilities that occur in graduate programs are often such that the disrespect or rudeness is subtle and is not always intended. This paper explores why graduate study presents a relatively high risk for incivilities, the kinds of incivilities that occur in graduate study, the effects incivilities have on the parties involved, and strategies for responding to and preventing incivilities in graduate programs.

Holly L. Mason, Ph.D., is Associate Dean and Professor, Purdue University School of Pharmacy, 1330 Heine Pharmacy Building, West Lafayette, IN 47906-1330 (E-mail: holly@pharmacy.purdue.edu).

[Haworth co-indexing entry note]: "Promoting Civility in Graduate Student Education." Mason, Holly L. Co-published simultaneously in *Journal of Pharmacy Teaching* (Pharmaceutical Products Press, an imprint of The Haworth Press, Inc.) Vol. 9, No. 3, 2002, pp. 57-70; and: *Promoting Civility in Pharmacy Education* (ed: Bruce A. Berger) Pharmaceutical Products Press, an imprint of The Haworth Press, Inc., 2003, pp. 57-70. Single or multiple copies of this article are available for a fee from The Haworth Document Delivery Service [1-800-HAWORTH, 9:00 a.m. - 5:00 p.m. (EST). E-mail address: docdelivery@haworthpress.com].

http://www.haworthpress.com/store/product.asp?sku=J060
© 2003 by The Haworth Press, Inc. All rights reserved.
10.1300/J060v09n03_05

UNDERSTANDING THE POTENTIAL FOR INCIVILITIES: THE NATURE OF GRADUATE STUDY

The graduate student is relatively powerless in the academic system. Graduate students must rely on the faculty to guide them through their educational experience. If a relationship with a faculty member turns bad, it could have lasting effects on the student's career. The faculty member might be the only person in a department who is able to facilitate completion of the student's degree program because of specialty area expertise. Further, the graduate student is dependent on the advisor to support applications for employment and, if the student ultimately obtains a position at an academic institution, he or she will most likely continue to encounter the former advisor throughout his or her career (2). This is particularly true in academic pharmacy where most of the faculty in a given discipline know each other well. A graduate student who runs afoul of some faculty member risks having to live with long-term consequences. Even with these dangers, faculty-graduate student relationships sometimes do go bad, often accompanied by very visible uncivil behaviors on the part of one or both parties.

Graduate study is stressful, in part, because of the power differential inherent in the academic system. Students entering a graduate program often have only a vague idea of what graduate school involves. They want to "do research" but do not know exactly what that means. Students rely on the faculty to guide them in this regard. Even students who have had extensive undergraduate research experience usually have not yet developed the ability to conceptualize and conduct research projects at the level required in graduate study. However, before students get to the stage in their program where they are able to become independent researchers, they need to confront the multiple responsibilities that graduate school presents. They are required to take challenging course loads, work as a graduate teaching assistant or a research assistant, and manage their personal and family life. Oftentimes these responsibilities coincide without the students having a good sense of how to get to where they want to go. This contributes to a sense of isolation that some graduate students feel during their program.

Graduate students are expected to develop independence, but they are dependent on an advisor to get them to that level. They are seen as more mature than undergraduate students, but the nature of graduate study is quite different from the undergraduate experience. Thus, the maturity needed to be successful at the graduate level cannot be assumed. Success in graduate study does not come only from taking a prescribed set of courses; it requires students to accept the open-ended time frame ubiquitous to the research process. Many students, when confronted with a task such as the dissertation, for which no end seems to be in sight, respond to their stress by demonstrating uncivil behaviors toward their faculty, their fellow students, and/or the undergraduate students they instruct.

Besides being relatively powerless and often under stress as they progress through their program, students must endure competition among themselves. This competition ranges from performance in courses to success in acceptances of abstracts and publications to recognition by faculty for their accomplishments. Although such competition can be healthy to some degree, it can become destructive if taken to extremes and may result in uncivil behavior among graduate students. Faculty members and specific features of a given graduate program can help keep stress and inappropriate competition at manageable levels. However, faculty members need to be careful that students do not become over reliant on them to solve the various routine problems and stresses faced by students during the course of graduate study.

WHAT TYPES OF INCIVILITIES OCCUR?

Numerous examples of incivilities can be cited. They are somewhat difficult to cleanly classify, as there are overlaps among them. However, listed below are examples of incivilities demonstrated by graduate students and faculty and incivilities that may be demonstrated by either. I have also commented on, as part of the section on graduate student incivility, incivilities in the classroom or teaching laboratory for which a graduate student has responsibility. Although examples of incivilities are provided, explicit solutions are not. In the subsequent section on "Preventing and Responding to Incivilities," suggestions are provided to address these problems.

Graduate Student Incivilities

Not Respecting Faculty Time. The student who does not show up for a scheduled appointment, the student who is chronically late for appointments, the student who abuses the faculty member's time by constantly extending the appointment with an effect on the faculty member's other responsibilities—these are all simple examples of not being respectful of the faculty member's time. Similarly, students who expect an unreasonably quick turnaround by the faculty member who is asked to review a proposal, a paper, or a data analysis are guilty of uncivil behavior. For a faculty member, the most frustrating situation occurs when the student demands that such a review be done that day because a proposal, project, or abstract is due the next day!

Not Meeting Responsibilities. There are a variety of manifestations of the graduate student not meeting his or her responsibilities. These include not performing tasks in a timely manner, doing incomplete or sloppy work, not making progress toward a degree objective, and neglecting one set of responsibilities for another (e.g., focusing on research and not performing acceptably as a teaching assistant). Because of the open-ended nature of graduate study, these kinds of behaviors can string out a program indefinitely if action is not taken to address the situation. This is particularly problematic if a graduate student is receiving financial support from a department, since willingness to fund a continuing student will affect the ability of the department to admit, support, and supervise new students.

Not Maintaining Quality Standards. Students sometimes do not realize that the faculty advisor is responsible for monitoring the accuracy, validity, and integrity of the student's research and for ensuring that the contributions of all participants in the research are properly acknowledged in disseminating the work. Students who submit abstracts or papers without review and oversight of a faculty member risk harming the reputation of their advisor and their department if problems are identified with the work. This kind of incivility is most often the result of the impatience of a student who wants to get the product of his or her efforts published quickly, without the recognition of the need for the quality control function played by the faculty advisor.

Plagiarism and Cheating. Outright cheating is relatively rare in graduate programs, but just as with undergraduate programs, graduate students who have previously taken a course do share papers, projects, and materials with students currently taking the class. This sometimes does provide opportunities for the student to make improper use of the shared materials. This same concern holds true for students working to develop thesis or dissertation proposals. There are also instances of occasional misconduct in terms of data fabrication or intentional misinterpretation of those data. In addition, just as with undergraduate study, there has been an increase in concerns about information obtained from the Internet. The vast amount of material available on the Internet is often inadequately referenced to begin with, and ease of retrieval make its use without adequate attribution tempting. And this is not just a problem related to the Internet. Sometimes graduate students are unwilling to make the effort to obtain original reference sources to properly reference and verify the accuracy of statements obtained through secondary sources.

Violence. Extreme examples of aggression by graduate students leading to the murder of university professors have been reported in the literature. Less extreme–but nonetheless troubling–student incivility includes physical assaults and threats made against the faculty (3). This kind of incivility is often the culmination of other, less severe incivilities. Thankfully, violence is seldom a problem in graduate programs, but it is something of which we need to be aware.

Graduate Students in the Classroom or Laboratory. Issues related to classroom incivility are not greatly different when the instructor is a graduate student or a professor, and this topic has been addressed by other authors in this issue. When a graduate student functions in the role of a teaching assistant, however, it is important to remember that he or she is not that far removed from the undergraduate experience. A typical teaching assistant has had little teaching experience and probably little instruction on how to teach. In general, they are similar to the students they are teaching. Because of their own role as a student they may tend to be more focused on their performance than on the needs of the students they are teaching.

Graduate students may be assigned to teach a course that is not in their direct area of expertise. Even faculty members have difficulty keeping up with content in their field that is not of day-to-day relevance to their work. Superficial knowledge about content, often combined with minimal teaching experience, can be an invitation to incivility by less mature undergraduate students. On the other hand, because of their limited classroom experience, graduate students are somewhat more prone to mistakes that even experienced faculty members sometimes make, such as handling sensitive subjects, inappropriate personal disclosure, and the handling of confidential information. Graduate students also need to be sensitive to misuse of power. Teaching assistants can respond to "being in charge" by abusing the power they have in making assignments, assigning grades, setting classroom policies, etc. They also must be aware of avoiding inappropriate romantic relationships with the students they teach. The potential for problems is sometimes magnified for international graduate students. International students often do not come from the same academic tradition, share the same educational values, or engage in the same communication style as students who are completing an undergraduate degree in this country.

Faculty Incivilities

Demonstrating Arrogance, Condescending Behaviors or Attitudes. Faculty sometimes fall into the trap of believing their superior experience and knowledge justifies conveying to students that they are only being tolerated and not respected as individuals with their own background knowledge and skills. This "overlord" attitude by faculty is easy to adopt given the relative powerlessness of graduate students, as discussed above. Abrupt or dismissive communication often goes hand-in-hand with arrogant or condescending behavior. Rather than listening to a student explain a problem or a plan, the faculty member may want to cut off the discussion and dictate to the student how the situation will be addressed. I have heard a faculty member say, "I don't want to hear any more about it. This is the way you will do it, if it is going to be done at all!"

Not Respecting a Student's Time. We have all encountered the case of a faculty member who, in an effort to encourage progress on a project, sets an unreasonable deadline for a student to complete the analysis of a data set. Although this strategy may be justifiable in the mind of the faculty member, it may be perceived by the graduate student to be an unfair, stress-producing task that he or she is being pressured to complete or suffer negative consequences. Other examples illustrating the faculty member not respecting the student's time include: frequently canceled appointments, constantly running late for appointments, not showing up at all for appointments, or not granting student appointments within a reasonable time frame. Neglecting to grade work or failing to comment on work in progress when promised shows disrespect for a student's time as well. Graduate students have multiple responsibilities. They need to be able to manage their time to complete a variety of tasks in a given week, ranging from course work, assigned projects, teaching assistant responsibilities, family responsibilities, and personal renewal time. Faculty members whose behaviors have a negative impact on this time management in a significant way are guilty of incivility.

Violating Academic Publication Traditions. Authorship disputes are potentially a major source of incivility in a graduate program. In many areas of research, it is not always clear who did what work or the most significant work on a study. When authorship credits are not clearly discussed in advance of publication, there is the real possibility of error. We have all heard of the professor who does not give authorship credit to the student who made a substantive contribution to a project, or worse, the faculty member who takes credit for the student's work and then unfairly omits the student's name from a research paper. Similarly, there are instances where an advisor may appropriate the ideas of a student to enhance the advisor's own reputation, thereby depriving the student of credit for the ideas. Scholarly activity and its dissemination are serious business in graduate programs. Both the faculty member and the student have much at stake when these kinds of disputes arise. If disputes are not handled appropriately, long-term harm can be done to both parties.

Abuse of Power. Consider the case of the graduate student who is assigned to teach a weekly laboratory section offered in conjunction with a larger lecture course. The student has the responsibility of developing a laboratory manual, setting up experiments, demonstrating the appropriate way to conduct the laboratory, and preparing and grading weekly quizzes. The student's advisor happens to be the instructor in charge of the course, and she asks the student to create slides for her lectures, write examination questions, and keep the grade book for the lecture portion of the course. The student is assigned to the course for ten hours a week, which is what is required to meet his assigned obligations. He finds that the additional tasks take up to 20 additional hours a week. This is certainly abuse of power on the part of the faculty member. Sometimes abuse of power is much less subtle. For example, expecting a graduate student to house-sit or baby-sit without pay is obviously an abuse of power. It becomes somewhat less clear when the faculty member asks the student to do outside tasks for pay. Does the student really have the opportunity to refuse the assignment?

Controlling Behavior. Controlling behavior is a more specific type of abuse of power. Sometimes a faculty member behaves in a way that denies a student the opportunity to make his or her own decisions. The faculty member who withholds information from a student about a grant opportunity or a summer internship because he believes the student would be better served focusing on his or her current research could be accused of incivility. Certainly, information is power, but that power is abused when it is used to control the student's behavior. The faculty member who refuses to forward letters of recommendation for certain job opportunities because the faculty member believes the positions are not a good "fit" for the student also demonstrates uncivil, controlling behavior.

Biased or Discriminating Behavior. Sometimes it appears that certain students, regardless of merit, receive more than their share of honors and opportunities in a graduate program. The problem is exacerbated when a given faculty member is advising multiple students but his or her "pet" student receives a disproportionate share of the rewards in terms of desirable teaching assignments, office or laboratory space, equipment, or opportunities to represent the department at various events or competitions. The appearance or reality is that some students are more valued than others in a program.

Joint Incivilities

Criticizing Faculty Members or Graduate Students. Making negative comments to fellow students or other faculty about the knowledge, skills, or behavior of a faculty member or student in a department or school may be considered uncivil behavior, particularly when the comments fail to provide the proper context for the comment. Sometimes when older students with experience in the field of study return to school, they are not shy about challenging their professor's knowledge about the applications of material. Although there is nothing wrong with doing so in a respectful manner, the utmost care on the part of the student is necessary to avoid the appearance of criticizing the knowledge of the faculty member. There is nothing as devastating to the morale of a department as public comments regarding abilities or behaviors of fellow department members.

Sharing Confidential Information. Both students and faculty members sometimes share personal or confidential information during their discussions. Students, in particular, often look to the faculty advisor as a source of advice regarding very personal matters that affect their work as graduate students. Students and faculty often assume that whatever is disclosed in meetings will be held in confidence (2). This is not necessarily true, and sometimes it is in the best interests of one or the other party to disclose certain types of information, depending upon the circumstances. Examples of these disclosures include issues that deal with student health and safety concerns, as well as gross violations of faculty or student behavioral standards. If ground rules have not been established between the faculty member and the student regarding information disclosure, it opens up the possibility of significant harm to one or both parties.

Displays of Anger. It is certainly not productive when a professor yells at a student or when a student displays the same behavior. This is true whether the interaction occurs when others are present or during private conversations. Even closed-door discussions that feature raised voices have a way of becoming known to others in the department. It does not help the faculty member-graduate student relationship when either displays anger in response to the perception that the other is "wrong." These displays are rightly viewed as degrading treatment, and incivility often begets further incivility.

Sexual Harassment or Misbehavior. Most universities have clear guidelines and policies related to sexual harassment or misbehavior, and the consequences to all parties involved can be significant. Beyond outright sexual misbehavior there are special risks in any sexual or romantic relationship between individuals in inherently unequal positions of power and authority. Such a relationship may undermine the integrity of the supervision and evaluation provided and may be less consensual than the individual whose position confers power believes it to be. Often such involvement may not even be recognized by the participants as inappropriate. However, such relationships certainly have the potential to harm others involved in the graduate program. The tensions involved in inappropriate relationships can affect the work of all others in a department who interact with the involved parties.

Incivilities Among Graduate Students

Many of the incivilities outlined previously similarly occur among graduate students. As noted, there is competitiveness among students in most graduate programs. In an attempt to "get ahead" of their fellow students or gain favor in the eyes of the graduate program faculty, students may be tempted to break the rules of civil behavior. The same strategies outlined in the subsequent section on preventing and responding to incivilities are relevant for these situations.

THE EFFECTS OF INCIVILITY
ON THE STUDENT AND FACULTY MEMBER

The effects of incivility on the student are numerous and interrelated. Professors are in a position to encourage or discourage their students by the style and content of their comments and interactions with the students. A faculty member can be hurtful in a number of ways, as discussed above. It is very difficult for a student to maintain a sense of self-worth during the process of becoming a genuine scholar (4). As a result, the student may experience a substantial loss in self-confidence, not only because of the power differential between the faculty member and the student, but because of the nature of the interactions. The loss of self-confidence and self-esteem often translates into a diminished productivity on the part of the student, and the student can lose sight of the goals that he or she has as a graduate student.

The faculty member experiencing incivilities may become frustrated, withdraw from normal mentoring responsibilities, and begin responding in a negative way to interactions with other graduate students and faculty colleagues. In the extreme, a faculty member can experience anxiety and fear for his or her safety.

PREVENTING AND RESPONDING TO INCIVILITIES

Making Expectations Known

It is important to send the message that each person within the graduate program community contributes to the success of the academic mission of the school, department, and university. Making expectations known is central to this success. A key to doing so is strong graduate program leadership. The individual or individuals responsible for the graduate program have a responsibility to make sure all students and faculty members involved in the program know what is expected of them and what behaviors are not to be tolerated. Graduate programs should have written policies and procedures that address areas where conflicts could arise. New students should be introduced to the policies, practices, and procedures of the department and university by means of an orientation session. A faculty advisor can be very effective in identifying areas of potential difficulty within a program without casting program policies or anticipated behaviors of colleagues in a negative light.

Students need to be regularly evaluated on their progress and performance. It is especially important for advisors to provide graduate students with timely and candid advice if their performance is deficient or if that performance might prevent them from attaining their degree objective. If the student is demonstrating uncivil behaviors, he or she needs to be told that those behaviors are unacceptable so the student has the opportunity to change. Similarly, the key to avoiding uncivil behavior in relation to teaching duties is teaching assistant training, supervision, and feedback.

Good Communication

It is important for the student's major professor to make a point of checking with the student frequently to see how things are going and to identify problems before they become major conflicts. It is important for the faculty member to always be polite and listen to students, even when he or she must turn down a request. The goal should be to work toward speaking with, rather than speaking at, the student. Graduate students may have difficulty turning down assignments or activities suggested by their advisor. It is important for the advisor to encourage the student to speak out if he or she begins to feel overloaded and, further, the advisor must make it clear that something can be done to address the problem. Both faculty and graduate students must be assertive enough to negotiate such things as deadlines and authorship of papers. Students should be encouraged to communicate concerns or questions to their advisor as soon as they arise. If difficulties are not addressed, they could get worse. Direct person-to-person communication should be used to solve problems. E-mails and memos should not be the first line of communication when problematic issues arise. The goal of direct communication is to avoid escalation of problems. Usually, difficulties can be worked out if both parties are willing to communicate. Sometimes a simple apology goes a long way toward resolving a conflict. When the faculty member–and/or the student–acknowledges how he or she has contributed to a problem and takes responsibility for it, there is a foundation for moving forward. Sometimes, despite efforts to work through problems, an inherent incompatibility between the student and the advisor becomes clear. In this case, a change of advisors may be in the interests of both parties.

Positive Role Modeling

Faculty must remember that they are role models for graduate students. Their approach to solving problems, their interaction style, and their response to conflict situations will be observed closely by the students with whom they interact. Faculty members can serve as positive role models for their faculty colleagues as well.

Major professors should recognize the existence of the power differential between themselves and their students and be sensitive to it. Faculty members need to realize that each student is unique, and they must respect and value the background and experience the student brings to interactions. Key traits that a faculty member can demonstrate as a positive role model include respect, patience, tolerance, compassion, sensitivity, and understanding.

One of the most important things a faculty member can do to prevent incivilities is to provide encouragement and reinforcement of positive behaviors. Graduate students respond to the positive comments and praise that their advisor provides. This goes a long way toward stimulating the kinds of behaviors desired in graduate students. It does not hurt to share with students appropriate disclosures about one's own positive and negative experiences as a graduate student. Again, this helps the student to visualize his or her own subsequent success in a program.

Maintaining Appropriate Boundaries

Some graduate students may actually be older or have more work experience in the field of study than the mentor or faculty. The close working relationship over time may result in the student misinterpreting the goals of the faculty member. Faculty members need to be careful to establish the boundaries of their working relationship with the student. There should be clear communication outlining the respective roles of the faculty member and student. The faculty member needs to make it clear that the relationship, although friendly, is strictly professional. This takes us back to the need for good communication between the graduate student and faculty member.

Hold People Responsible for Transgressions

If someone violates standards, action must be taken to hold him or her accountable or no real progress will be achieved. Often penalties for significant transgressions are specified in written policies. These penalties could range from loss of certain privileges to withdrawal of financial support to dismissal from the program. There should be an established procedure for putting the student (or a faculty member) on notice that particular behaviors will not be tolerated. Subsequent violation of the policy or a repeat of the behavior should result in previously specified penalties. Faculty have a responsibility to prevent inappropriate behaviors from continuing. They need to call attention to consequences of violating standards and to encourage students to think carefully before they speak and to avoid emotive or inflammatory language.

Have an Effective Grievance Process

To prevent graduate student-faculty or graduate student-professional program student conflict from escalating, a process must be in place wherein student complaints and concerns are taken seriously and appropriately investigated. It is not unusual for the aggrieved party to complain that his or her concerns are trivialized or dismissed offhand. Most institutions have a grievance process in place. Such a process typically asks the parties involved to go through a chain of command such that if the parties cannot work out their conflict, discussion moves to the next higher level (an advisor, course director, program director, or department chair) for conflict resolution. The formal grievance process should be viewed as a last resort if a problem cannot be resolved. An intermediary step that can often be effective is the ombudsperson. Many universities have established ombudsperson offices in recent years. An ombudsperson is an impartial, independent, and confidential resource for helping to resolve conflicts or misunderstandings. Whether disputes are resolved informally or formally, there must be clear communication to all parties regarding resolution of the problem and safeguards should be put in place to prevent a recurrence of the situation.

CONCLUSION

Incivility in graduate education can have a deleterious effect on students, faculty, and the entire educational process. The nature and structure of graduate study is such that incivility can flourish unless mechanisms are in place to prevent it. Graduate education is conducted in a high-stress environment: the professional career of the graduate student and career advancement for the faculty member are at stake, at least to some extent.

Encouragement of civil behavior begins by having a shared set of expectations for behavior of graduate students and faculty members involved in a program. Shared expectations can then be reinforced by clear and frequent communication among graduate program participants. Success in expectation setting and effective communications is usually a function of strong graduate program leadership. Faculty members have an opportunity to further reinforce the behavioral standards of a graduate program by personally modeling the positive behavioral characteristics they expect of their colleagues and graduate students. When uncivil behaviors do occur, steps need to be taken to address them and the party or parties involved must be held responsible for their behavior. The existence of effective informal and formal grievance process features can facilitate resolution of disputes stemming from uncivil behavior.

The presence of the graduate program features enumerated above will increase the satisfaction of both faculty and graduate students involved with the program. If one begins with the goal of having all parties demonstrate positive, civil behaviors in all aspects of their graduate program participation and there are mechanisms in place to encourage and enforce these behaviors, the need to address uncivil behaviors will be minimal.

REFERENCES

1. Berger BA. Promoting civility in pharmacy education: Introduction. *J Pharm Teach.* 2002; 9(3):1-10.

2. Prieto LR, Meyers SA. The teaching assistant training handbook. Stillwater, OK: New Forums Press; 2001.

3. Morrissette PJ. Reducing incivility in the university/college classroom. *Int Electron J Leadership Learn.* 2001; 5(4). Available at http://www.ucalgary.ca/~iejll/volume5/morrissette.html.

4. Arnstein RL, et al. Helping students adapt to graduate school: Making the grade. New York: The Haworth Press, Inc.; 2000.

Civility and Professionalism

Dana P. Hammer

INTRODUCTION

Professionalism is a topic that has received a fair amount of attention in recent years in health professions education. And, with this collection devoted specifically to civility in pharmacy education, it seems appropriate to look at the relationship between professionalism and civility. The concepts of professionalism and civility certainly seem interrelated, if not equal on some levels, and as a reader of these types of articles, you might be asking yourself, "What exactly is the difference between civility and professionalism?" Although there is much overlap between these two concepts, there are distinct differences as well. This article will explore the relationship between civility and professionalism, discuss approaches to handling incivilities and unprofessional behavior, and provide strategies for cultivating civility and professionalism in our students.

THE RELATIONSHIP BETWEEN CIVILITY AND PROFESSIONALISM

This section begins with a discussion of the complex concept of professionalism to clarify the distinction between it and civility. *Merriam-*

Dana P. Hammer, Ph.D., R.Ph., is Director of the Bracken Pharmaceutical Care Learning Center and University of Washington Community Pharmacy Residency Program, University of Washington School of Pharmacy, Box 357630, Seattle, WA 98195-7630.

[Haworth co-indexing entry note]: "Civility and Professionalism." Hammer, Dana P. Co-published simultaneously in *Journal of Pharmacy Teaching* (Pharmaceutical Products Press, an imprint of The Haworth Press, Inc.) Vol. 9, No. 3, 2002, pp. 71-90; and: *Promoting Civility in Pharmacy Education* (ed: Bruce A. Berger) Pharmaceutical Products Press, an imprint of The Haworth Press, Inc., 2003, pp. 71-90. Single or multiple copies of this article are available for a fee from The Haworth Document Delivery Service [1-800-HAWORTH, 9:00 a.m. - 5:00 p.m. (EST). E-mail address: docdelivery@haworthpress.com].

http://www.haworthpress.com/store/product.asp?sku=J060
© 2003 by The Haworth Press, Inc. All rights reserved.
10.1300/J060v09n03_06

Webster's Collegiate Dictionary gives one definition of professionalism as "the conduct, aims, or qualities that characterize or mark a professional or a professional person" (1). The "White Paper on Pharmacy Student Professionalism" defined it as "the active demonstration of the traits of a professional" (2). Others have described professionalism as "constituting those attitudes and behavior that serve to maintain patient interest above [physician] self-interest," and "displaying values, beliefs and attitudes that put the needs of another above your personal needs" (3, 4). It has also been written that:

> Professionalism is displayed in the way pharmacists conduct themselves in professional situations. This definition implies a demeanor that is created through a combination of behaviors, including courtesy and politeness when dealing with patients, peers, and other health care professionals. Pharmacists should consistently display respect for others and maintain appropriate boundaries of privacy and discretion. Whether dealing with patients or interacting with others on a health care team, it is important to possess–and display–an empathetic manner. (5)

Although these definitions of professionalism are given mostly in terms of attitudes and specific behaviors of professionals, the origin of the concept was based on somewhat different attributes. Social science literature of the 1950s and 1960s defined professionalism based on the possession of certain characteristics: professions and professionals possess sets of *structural* and *attitudinal* attributes that distinguish them from occupations and members thereof (6-11). Structural attributes of professions and professionals include:

- Specialized body of knowledge and skills
- Unique socialization of student members
- Licensure/certification
- Professional associations
- Governance by peers
- Social prestige
- Vital service to society
- Code of ethics
- Autonomy
- Equivalence of members
- Special relationship with clients.

Attitudinal attributes of professionals were described as:

- Use of the professional organization as a major reference, i.e., using professional colleagues as the major source of professional ideas and judgments in practice
- Belief in service to the public, i.e., one's professional practice is indispensable to society and benefits the public
- Belief in self-regulation, i.e., one's peers are the best qualified to judge one's work
- Sense of calling to the field, i.e., dedication to the profession regardless of extrinsic rewards
- Autonomy, i.e., one can make professional decisions without external pressures from clients, nonprofessionals, and employers.

Thus, upon review of the literature we can determine that professionalism is a complex composite of structural, attitudinal, and behavioral attributes. No wonder the concept is so broadly used and widely interpreted by professionals, members of occupations, and consumers in any given society! A broader definition of professionalism that attempted to encompass all of the aforementioned characteristics was offered by this author in a previous paper: "[Professionalism] is the possession and/or demonstration of structural, attitudinal and behavioral attributes of a profession and its members" (12).

To contrast this definition with that of civility, we turn once again to *Merriam-Webster's Collegiate Dictionary*, where civility is defined as: "1 *archaic*: training in the humanities, 2 a: courtesy, politeness b: a polite act or expression" (13). Definitions 2a and 2b seem most applicable to our current discussion. These definitions of civility could be categorized as *behavioral* attributes of professionalism; thus, civility is a *component* of professionalism.

If we think more broadly about the concept of civility, however, civility could be considered a basic set of accepted behaviors for a society/culture upon which professional behaviors are rooted. In other words, civility must be present to have professionalism. It is the minimum set of standards for professional behavior; it serves as the foundation for professionalism (Figure 1). We would expect most members of a given culture or society to exhibit at least civil behaviors, but more "professional" members of that society/culture would be expected to consistently exhibit civil behaviors as well as professional behaviors. For example, communicating articulately, relating empathically, practicing ethically, exceeding expectations, and putting others' needs above

FIGURE 1

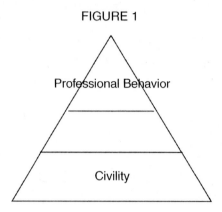

one's own might be considered professional behaviors–they go beyond what we might consider civil behaviors. A society/culture may not expect all of its citizens to demonstrate the aforementioned behaviors, but it may expect its members to demonstrate, at minimum, respect toward one another, for example.

Another way to describe the relationship between civil and professional behavior is to examine the *frequency with which* and *degree to which* civil behaviors are demonstrated. A more "professional" person would be expected to demonstrate civil behaviors more often and to a greater degree than a nonprofessional person–behaviors such as respect, politeness, and courtesy. Societies desire to hold their professionals to higher standards of behaviors. To illustrate this, just think of how much media attention is devoted to a professional person if that person demonstrates unprofessional behavior (e.g., Bill Clinton, O. J. Simpson, Jim Baker).

Although a clear distinction between civility and professionalism may still not be evident, suffice it to say that without civility there cannot be professionalism. Professionalism is civility at a "higher" level–exceeding expectations versus meeting them. Also, one may be civil in attempting to get one's own needs met, but the same behavior may be unprofessional. As an example, a pharmacist may politely and respectfully give a patient her medication without any counseling. This would be civil, yet unprofessional due to professional codes of conduct. It is important to remember that civil and professional behaviors are defined by society, culture, and generations. Thus, what is considered civil or professional in one culture may not necessarily be considered civil or professional in others. This is easily illustrated if you think in terms of generational values: what is considered acceptable and appropriate changes as we advance in age. It is perfectly acceptable to Generation X to have a pierced eyebrow, while the grandparents of Generation X find the same practice offensive and unprofessional. Thus, the relationship between civility and professionalism may differ, depending on a society's values.

APPROACHES TO HANDLING INCIVILITIES AND UNPROFESSIONAL BEHAVIORS

This section describes "macro" approaches for handling incivilities and unprofessional behaviors such as the negative behavior/punitive approach, positive behavior/reward approach, a combination approach, and the "do nothing" approach. This section also discusses methods for establishing which approach or approaches will be used in a given course or institution. Other articles in this volume discuss more specific response strategies depending on the negative behavior demonstrated.

Negative Behavior → Punitive Approach

"Bad dog" (13). The basic tenet of this approach is that a subject should be punished for demonstrating an undesirable behavior. The source of motivation, then, for subjects *not* to participate in these behaviors is that there is punishment involved. This approach is usually practiced in societies and cultures where the "norm" or minimum expectation(s) is/are always expected to be met. Action occurs only when an assumption or norm is violated. Consider the case of pharmacy education. Unwritten expectations/assumptions of our students are that they will act as mature adults, value their education, and treat others with respect. Thus, when a student is caught cheating, there is a punishment involved. The clerkship student who consistently arrives at the practice site late and unprepared is marked down on the clerkship evaluation form. These students are usually the 10% (or less) who consume 90% of a faculty member's time (tongue in cheek). With the negative-punitive approach, guidelines or minimum expectations are not always explicitly articulated to the population; they are simply assumed to be known.

Positive Behavior → Reward Approach

"Good dog" (13). The basic tenet of this approach is that a subject is rewarded when it demonstrates a desired behavior. The source of motivation, then, for subjects to demonstrate these behaviors is that there is a reward involved. This is not to say that the only time subjects demonstrate the desired behaviors is when there is a reward involved, but it can serve as the motivating factor for some subjects. This approach is usually practiced in cultures where the "norm" is that of *not* meeting or exceeding expectations for behavior, so a reward system is established to create motivation for them to do so. Consider the case of an alternative education program for convicted juvenile offenders. Because many of the offenders may not consider education important, instructors may offer field trips, prizes, or bonus points to those students who choose to have perfect attendance in class. In pharmacy education, the "good dog" approach may be illustrated as scholarships, "A" grades (although some students *expect* to receive A's), extra credit, a day off from class, and other rewards. With the positive-reward approach, goals and expectations are usually defined so that students know what the "target" is and what they need to do to attain the reward.

Combination and "Do Nothing" Approaches

Most educational programs use a combination of the negative and positive approaches to avoid negative behaviors and promote positive ones, although these approaches may not always be explicitly articulated as such. However, in the past there may not have seemed as great a need to establish punitive and reward systems to help govern behavior in educational programs. It was "known" that education was a privilege, not a right, and that hard work was expected to learn as much as possible and take advantage of the opportunity to be educated. Educational programs in the past may have subconsciously employed the "do nothing" approach. There was no need to punish undesirable behavior or reward positive behavior because the norm was that all subjects met and/or exceeded expectations to the level of their ability.

TOP-DOWN OR BOTTOM-UP:
WHICH APPROACH IS MOST SUCCESSFUL?

The process of establishing guidelines for behavior and its subsequent punishment or reward is fundamental in guiding a system's success or failure. Consider the first year, first semester pharmacy class. Because these students are unfamiliar with the school's program, it is appropriate for the faculty and administration to design and implement guidelines for expected behaviors. These are then presented and made explicit to students so that there is no question what the school expects of them. On the other end of the continuum, as these students progress through the program and become more mature students (some mature to a higher level and faster than others), it may be appropriate to let *them* determine what the expectations for their behavior should be and how it should be rewarded and/or punished, if at all. The latter idea supports principles of adult education and also illustrates the concept of "buy in"–if they help create it, they are more likely to support/abide by it.

Consider the example of the Professional Skills Development course sequence at the University of Colorado Health Sciences Center School of Pharmacy. In the first semester of the first year, the course instructors determine the dress code for the course and the consequences of not adhering to the dress code. In the second year of the course sequence, the instructors make minor modifications to the dress code with students' input. The third year of the course has students determining their own dress code. Lo and behold, it looks amazingly similar to the codes from previous years. The students have matured professionally enough to understand the importance of a dress code and to appreciate the respect, trust, and level of responsibility that the instructors show them as they have progressed through the program. This maturation process has, in part, been facilitated by the instructors having previously set guidelines and provided a reasonable expectation why these guidelines exist.

It is difficult to determine whether the former, "top-down" approach or the latter, "bottom-up" approach is more successful when establishing and implementing expectation and consequence systems. Programs that use faculty/student committees to establish and/or enforce codes of conduct may choose to employ a combination of approaches. Acceptance and impact will depend on the students' level of responsibility and maturity with the given system.

CULTIVATING CIVILITY/PROFESSIONALISM IN OUR STUDENTS

This section explores general ideas of how educators may develop, maintain, and improve the behavior of their students. For additional guidelines and more specific ideas, refer to other articles in this work, the "White Paper on Pharmacy Student Professionalism," and a previously referenced paper (2, 12).

Recruitment and Admissions

For the most part, educators know that it is easier to teach students a subject or skill if the students already possess some knowledge of or have previous experience with that subject or skill. Intuitively, then, we know it should be easier to develop, maintain, and improve students' professional behavior if they come into our programs already possessing some of the desired traits. What kinds of students are we recruiting? How can we focus our attention on those students who already demonstrate civil and professional behaviors? Is there a way we could communicate with the counselors and faculty in our "feeder" programs so that they could encourage students with these traits, among others, to apply to our programs? Interaction with the prepharmacy majors on our campuses can also help us to identify those applicants who may demonstrate desired traits more than others. Are students who demonstrate active participation (versus membership just to get the résumé item) in the school's prepharmacy club given more consideration in the application process? Service to the profession is certainly a desirable professional trait.

What about our recruiting materials and presentations? Do we discuss the kinds of desired traits and behaviors that pharmacists and pharmacy students should possess? Reviewing and modifying these materials for this sort of content may be a beneficial exercise that may result in attracting desirable students.

Most admissions processes in schools of pharmacy include the collection of recommendation letters from various sources who know the applicant, as well as on-site interviews to help determine candidates' communication ability, demeanor, and general social skills. But even with these activities, we know that programs still admit students who later on show their "true colors"–very different behavior from what was demonstrated in their interviews or what was stated in their recommendation letters. So how can we gather more accurate data about these students before they enter our programs? I do not have a good answer to this question, but I have been thinking about more rigorous screening methods where we could contact previous employers, instructors, or colleagues of interviewees via telephone to ask specific questions about the applicant. Of course this would be a time-intensive process that would add even more hours to an already time-intensive process. But perhaps the knowledge gained from an information-seeking process like this could save the school more time and energy later.

Admissions committees should consider having applicants complete standardized instruments that have predictive potential for student success and other parameters. For example, Rest's Defining Issues test has been shown to be a predictor of cognitive moral development and clinical performance (14, 15). Although a full discussion of predictive instruments is beyond the scope of this article, there is an abundance of literature in pharmacy education that describes them.

Programmatic–Culture, Curriculum, and Extra-Curriculum

Within our programs, there are a number of areas in which we can devote attention to help foster professionalism in our students. Examine the culture and environment of your program. Are the policies employed conducive to fostering professional behavior of students, administrators, faculty, preceptors, teaching assistants, staff, and others with whom students come into contact? For example, maybe there is a policy of no cell phones allowed during class without prior permission of the instructor. In addition to an honor code, are there policies regarding other specific unprofessional behaviors or incivilities? If so, are these policies used and enforced? Are there consequences for the student who consistently violates these codes? Additionally, are the policies that are meant for students applicable to faculty? If so, are those enforced? We often have guidelines that explicate what is expected of students, but do we have similar documents concerning what students should expect of faculty? Professional development requires mentoring and, more importantly, role modeling.

Targeted faculty development can also help to reduce negative behaviors in our programs. Do all faculty members, especially new faculty members, participate in educational programs about how to promote civility and professionalism in the classroom and minimize or prevent incivilities? Are there mentors, guidelines, or other sources of support where faculty members can go for advice?

What about the facilities of your school of pharmacy? Are they clean, are they organized, and do they present a professional image? Are the classrooms, supplies, and equipment well kept and up to date? A professional physical environment can go a long way in helping to maintain a positive professional atmosphere for students and faculty.

Educators can also employ strategies within courses that help develop students' professionalism. One way is to establish behavioral policies, such as the cell phone example above, that are peripheral to course content. Another way is to create activities and assignments that focus on professional behavior and professionalism as a part of the course content. Consider once again our colleagues at the University of Colorado Health Sciences Center School of Pharmacy. In the Professional Skills Development course sequence, students evaluate themselves on their professional behavior periodically, meet with a faculty member to discuss their assessment, and then develop a written professional plan for improving their weaknesses and maintaining their strengths (Appendix A). In subsequent meetings with faculty members, students discuss their progress and modify their plans if needed. Faculty members also provide input about the student's professional behavior based on their observations of the student. Peer assessment is employed as part of the courses. Although a single course, or even a series of courses, cannot be completely responsible for students' professional development, such courses can certainly go a long way in helping students (and faculty) to define professional behavior and foster its development.

Another way to approach professionalism and civility within the classroom is to make behavioral evaluation part of students' grades or requirements to pass the course. This could be considered either a negative-punitive approach or a positive-reward approach, depending on how it is established. For example, if a student is consistently tardy to class, that student's grade is adversely affected. These policies can be successful as long as the behavioral expectations and grading system are made explicit to students and there are valid methods for documenting students' behavior.

Most experiential programs already employ some sort of behavioral evaluation of students. These behavioral criteria should be reviewed to make sure that they are specific and consistently interpreted the same way by preceptors. For example, the line item on an evaluation form "Student displays professional behavior" is much more vague and open to various interpretations than specific items like "Student is prompt and punctual," "Student adheres to dress code employed by the practice site," and "Student is respectful toward patients, supervisors, staff, and other health care professionals." Of course, the more specific the evaluation becomes, the lengthier and more time-consuming it becomes. When reviewing these behavioral criteria, one also needs to ask about the weight given to these items versus the skill-based or competency items. If all items on an evaluation form are given equal weight and there are 25 skill-based items and 3 behavioral items, then it seems that there is not much value placed on the behaviors.

Lastly, professionalism and professional behavior can be fostered in extracurricular activities. Are students encouraged to serve as representatives of the school to their community? Do they get involved with local agencies and organizations? Are the student organizations more than just social and party groups? Are the advisors for the groups serving as positive professional role models? Positive involvement in extracurricular activities helps to develop students' structural and attitudinal characteristics of professionalism as well as the behavioral aspects of professionalism.

CONCLUSION

If we consider civility to be an accepted set of behaviors that maintains the decorum of a given society or culture and professionalism to be the possession and/or demonstration of structural, attitudinal, and behavioral attributes of a profession and its members, the relationship between the two concepts can be described as this: civility serves as the foundation upon which professional behavior is rooted, and professional behavior is part of the complex concept of professionalism.

Approaches to handling incivilities and unprofessional behavior can be classified into four categories: negative-punitive approach, positive-reward approach, a combination of the two, or "do nothing." There are many areas that schools can address to promote civil and professional behavior and to minimize undesirable behaviors: recruitment/admissions, programmatic policies and procedures, physical environment, faculty development, classroom activities, assignments and grading policies, the experiential program, and extracurricular activities. As schools pay more attention to students' behavioral development in addition to their knowledge and skill development, we should hope to see student behavior improving or, at least, not worsening.

REFERENCES

1. Merriam-Webster's Collegiate Dictionary. 10th ed. Springfield, MA: Merriam-Webster Inc.; 1997.

2. APhA-ASP/AACP-COD Task Force on Professionalism. White paper on pharmacy student professionalism. *J Am Pharm Assoc.* 2000; 40(1):96-102.

3. American Board of Internal Medicine. Project professionalism. Philadelphia: American Board of Internal Medicine; 1995.

4. Beardsley RS. Chair report of the APhA-ASP/AACP-COD Task Force on Professionalization: Enhancing professionalism in pharmacy education and practice. *Am J Pharm Educ.* 1996; 60(Winter Suppl):26S-28S.

5. Chalmers RK. Contemporary issues: Professionalism in pharmacy. *Tomorrow's Pharm.* 1997; (Mar):10-12.

6. Parsons T. The social system. Glencoe, IL: The Free Press; 1951.

7. Greenwood E. Attributes of a profession. *Soc Work.* 1957; 2(Jul):44-55.

8. Strauss G. Professionalism and occupational associations. *Ind Rel.* 1963; 2(3):8-9.

9. Wilensky HL. The professionalization of everyone? *Am J Sociol.* 1964; 70: 137-46.

10. Vollmer HM, Mills DL, eds. Professionalization. 1st ed. Englewood Cliffs, NJ: Prentice-Hall, Inc.; 1966.

11. Hall RH. Professionalization and bureaucratization. *Am Sociol Rev.* 1968; 33(Feb):92-104.

12. Purkerson Hammer D. Professional attitudes and behaviors: The "A's and B's" of professionalism. *Am J Pharm Educ.* 2000; 64:455-64.

13. Paulsen S. Personal communication, May 2001.

14. Latif D. Moral reasoning: Should it serve as a criterion for student and resident selection in pharmacy? *Am J Pharm Educ.* 2001; 65:119-24.

15. Latif D, et al. Relationship between community pharmacists' moral reasoning and components of clinical performance. *J Soc Admin Pharm.* 1998; 15:210-24.

APPENDIX A

PHRD 3100: Professional Skills Development I
Fall 2000

Course Directors:

Dana Hammer, Ph.D.	Susan Paulsen, Pharm.D.
Assistant Professor	Assistant Professor
Office: 352	Office: 354C

office hours by appointment

(o) 303-315-0701	(o) 303-315-8427
(f) 303-315-4630	(p) 303-599-1787
dana.hammer@uchsc.edu	susan.paulsen@uchsc.edu

Teaching Assistants:

Yvonne Lentz	Lori Girouard
yvonne.lentz@uchsc.edu	lorinda.girouard@uchsc.edu

Disclaimer: *This syllabus is a living, breathing document and will be referred to throughout the course. The course directors reserve the right to add, remove, and/or modify portions of it throughout the semester. **The integrative nature of this course lends itself to flexibility in scheduling activities. As uncomfortable as this is for students and faculty, it is a necessary feature to maintain the quality of the course.** Students, other involved faculty and teaching assistants will be notified immediately if/when changes are made.*

Required Materials:
Necessary preparation for each session
Positive attitude and professional behavior
Respect for self and others
Willingness to learn
Flexibility
Student ID
White lab coat (see page 7)
Professional attire (see page 7)
Calculator
Internet access
University email account

Required Text: Khan, MA, and Reddy, IK. Pharmaceutical and Clinical Calculations, Ed. 2, Technomic Publishing Co., Lancaster, PA. (ISBN 1-56676-812-8)

Access of Materials and Information: In addition to what you are provided in class, materials and information will be distributed using:
1) Blackboard® (http://bullwinkle/courses/PHRD3100/), an electronic education delivery system. Students will receive instruction on enrollment and access during orientation.
2) your school email account.
These systems are **mandatory** communications modalities among faculty and students for this course. Most materials will be able to be accessed a week prior to the module via these systems.

APPENDIX A (continued)

Educational Philosophies *(aka "the world according to Drs. Hammer and Paulsen")*:

This course was designed based on the assumptions that students **want to learn** about the profession of pharmacy, will **actively participate** in learning activities, and **work to achieve their potential**. In turn, the course directors, other involved faculty and teaching assistants will create a learning environment to facilitate operationalization of this philosophy. This course is also based on the educational philosophies of **mastery learning** and **assessment-as-learning** to help students achieve course outcomes.

Mastery learning is demonstrated as individual students achieve the outcomes and competencies of a particular course or project. If students can demonstrate such achievement, then they earn the "grade" associated with that achievement. By contrast, courses that operate using a "norm-referenced" philosophy compare an individual student's achievement to other students' achievements and attempt to create a normalized distribution of students based on their level of achievement. Thus, many norm-referenced graded courses have bell-shaped distributions of students' grades while many mastery learning-graded courses may have large numbers of students on the higher end of the grading scale, similar to graduate-level courses.

Assessment-as-learning is a concept originally described by Alverno College in Milwaukee, Wisconsin. It incorporates the notion that feedback provided to students regarding their performance on a particular exercise, for example, helps them to determine their strengths and weaknesses in relation to that exercise so that they can improve performance when reassessed. The concept can also be interpreted to mean that the assessment methods associated with a particular course or project will "drive" the manner in which students learn – especially in a graded system. For example, if a course utilizes performance on knowledge-based exams as the primary method of assessment of student learning, then students can be expected to memorize and regurgitate the knowledge on which they are being tested. By contrast, if a course assesses students' learning using performance on knowledge-based exams in addition to writing papers, making oral presentations, or participating in class discussions, then students could be expected to memorize and regurgitate knowledge, write content relevant, grammatically correct papers, make effective oral presentations or actively participate in class discussions. In other words, students will usually perform in the manner in which they are incited.

Course Description: This one-semester course is the first in a five-semester longitudinal course sequence intended to develop a broad range of skills necessary for **current** and **future** pharmacy practice. It is designed to parallel the didactic portion of the curriculum, integrating and applying essential knowledge, skills and attitudes required for a successful professional career.

Uniquely, this course lends continuity and cohesiveness to the entire curriculum. Each year, as students assemble their pharmacy knowledge base, the Professional Skills course gives students the opportunity to integrate information within a given semester and from semester-to-semester. Additionally, students will be able and expected to practice and refine a variety of skills through collaborative and individual activities. As this course builds over three years of the curriculum, students will be able to observe and document their own progression towards achievement of professional, academic and personal goals.

Course Outcomes: Upon completion of the Fall P1 semester, the student is expected to be able to:

1. Identify one's own and other's strengths and weaknesses as a communicator on the interpersonal level.
2. Identify and develop methods of verbal, non-verbal, and written communication in a variety of situations.
3. Demonstrate the ability to utilize the campus informatics system to achieve module and course outcomes.
4. Demonstrate the ability to document accurate information and provide evidence for decision-making.
5. Demonstrate accurate observational, comprehension, and evaluative skills.
6. Utilize problem-solving processes to resolve pharmacy-related issues.
7. Identify one's own personal, cultural, and generational values in the context of professional situations.
8. Recognize and effectively utilize one's own behaviors while involved in teamwork/group activities.
9. Identify behaviors, both personal and other's, that support or detract from professionalism.
10. Demonstrate expected professional and classroom behavior as outlined in the School's Student Ethics and Conduct Code and the Professional Behavior Assessment Form.
11. Effectively utilize and integrate knowledge from concurrent and prior courses and experiences to solve problems presented in class.

Course Schedule: This 3-credit course meets weekly every Monday and Wednesday, from 2:00 - 5:00 p.m., and Friday, from 1:00 – 4:00 p.m. (except for Monday August 28th which is rescheduled to meet Tuesday August 29th from 2:00-5:00 p.m. and Monday September 4th which is rescheduled to meet on Wednesday September 6th from 7:30 – 10:30 a.m). Class is cancelled Friday November 24th for the Thanksgiving holiday. Students from this Friday section will be rescheduled for earlier in the Thanksgiving week. Each student is assigned to one specific 3-hour section per week.

Course Feedback: Students will have the opportunity to provide the course directors, instructors and teaching assistants with course feedback in several ways:

- make appointment with course director(s)
- talk with class representative(s) who report to course directors' meetings (anonymity of persons making comments is maintained with student representatives)
- a mid-semester course-specific evaluation
- a formal university-wide evaluation process at the end of the semester

Policy Information

Class Decorum: This is a *PROFESSIONAL* Skills course. Students are expected to behave and perform as professionals-in-training, *i.e.*, demonstrate respect for course instructors, their peers and themselves; participate in all course activities with purpose and a positive attitude; and abide by course policies. Eating during laboratory activities, reading the newspaper, working on other courses' material, or other activities that distract from course activities are not allowed. Additionally, the use of cellular phones and pagers will not be allowed without the prior consent of the course directors. Because professional behavior is so important for persons entering an established profession, **your behavior during the course will be observed and periodically evaluated by faculty** and teaching

APPENDIX A (continued)

assistants using the Professional Behavior Assessment (PBA) form. You will be given the opportunity to **assess yourself** using the same instrument and discuss your assessment with course directors. A specified number of points toward your final grade will be allocated for the assessment of your professional behavior based on the faculty and teaching assistants' observations.

Assessment Policy: *Assessment* differs from *evaluation*. Assessment includes **feedback** that is used for the purpose of **improving** one's performance; evaluation is used to assign a grade or make a decision. In this course, assessors of your classroom performance will include yourself, your peers, standardized patients, instructors and teaching assistants. The nature and point value of assessments will vary weekly depending upon the type and complexity. These issues will be presented and discussed in the week prior to the assessment(s), if not before.

This course is subject to two levels of evaluation. The first relates to allocation of letter grades wherein grades are based on the total number of points accumulated by a student in the course. The second level of evaluation involves demonstration of mastery learning, i.e., a student must pass all assignments. It is important for the student to understand that he/she can receive a grade of "IF" independently of his/her point score, i.e., if a student fails an assignment or skill, they will receive an "IF" for the course.

Requirements for Passing this Course: In order to pass the course (C- or better), students must achieve all course outcomes. This entails students completing and passing all assignments, quizzes and exams. Failure to meet these expectations will result in a grade of **IF (Incomplete failure)**.

Grading Policy: Each Professional Skills Development 3-hour session will be worth a minimum of 25 but no more than 75 points. The final grade for this course will be assigned as a percentage of the total allowable points attained (percentages will be rounded as necessary). The percentage will then be converted to a letter grade according to the following University of Colorado Health Sciences Center grading scale:

93-100%	A	83-86	B	73-76%	C
90-92	A-	80-82	B-	69.5-72	C-
87-89	B+	77-79	C+	< 69.45	IF

Minimum passing grade for this course is **C-** (refer to "Academic Standing" section of the Student Handbook).

Quizzes and Exams:
Quizzes and exams may involve performance-based assessments in addition to short answer and multiple choice questions. Performance-based assessment examples include completing a task on the computer, utilizing drug information resources to answer questions, telephone activities, and compounding. **All calculations are considered to be either correct or incorrect; no partial credit will be given.** Calculations with misplaced decimal points, mislabeled or unlabeled units, unmeasurable quantities, inappropriate zero placement or inappropriate rounding will be considered incorrect and no credit will be given. Failure to show your work is considered an incorrect answer; as such, no credit will be given under these circumstances.

Quizzes: There will be two cumulative quizzes (see below) worth 50 points each. Additional quizzes, announced and/or unannounced may also be given in class on assigned readings.

QUIZ #1   October 4   8:00-10:00am   *Vincent and Gutke* modules 1-5   **50 points**

QUIZ #2   November 6 8:00-10:00am   *Vincent and Gutke* modules 6-10   **50 points**

Exam: There will be one cumulative final exam (date TBA) worth 100 points.

FINAL EXAM	modules 1-5	25%	**100 points**
	modules 6-10	25%	
	modules 11-16	50%	

Expectations for Assignments:
Students will be expected to demonstrate skills and attributes of a developing professional. Students are expected to complete each assignment following the provided instructions. Students failing to follow the instructions will have their papers returned ungraded. These assignments must be resubmitted within one week and will receive a maximum of half the original possible points. Assignments handed in late **will receive zero points** unless prior consent is obtained from course directors.
Expectations for calculations are described in Exams and Quizzes and pertain to all assignments. All electronic assignments must be submitted in Microsoft Word®.

Other Assessments:
Patient Consultation: There will be one baseline assessment (25 points), one midterm (50 points), and one final (100 points) patient consultation videotaped exercise (to be completed at Belle Bonfils with standardized patients– see dates in course calendar).
Peer and Self-Assessment for Team Behaviors: There will be one (50 point) mid-term peer and self-assessment and one final peer and self-assessment of team behavior (50 points).
Professionalism Self and Faculty Assessment: Students will have an individual meeting with one of the course directors twice during the semester to discuss professional behaviors. In addition, students will be required to write two short papers (graded for content and grammar) and complete three self-assessments. Fifty points will be assigned to the first paper/first meeting and 100 points to second paper /second meeting.

TABLE OF POINTS

ASSESSMENT	MINIMUM POINTS	MAXIMUM POINTS
TWO QUIZZES AND FINAL EXAM	200	200
(UN)ANNOUNCED QUIZZES	0	100
PATIENT CONSULTATION	175	175
PEER/SELF-ASSESSMENTS	100	100
PROFESSIONALISM ASSESSMENT	150	150
WEEKLY MODULES	14 weeks x 25 points = 350	10 weeks x 25 points and 4 weeks x 75 points = 550
TOTAL POINTS	**975 POINTS**	~~1375~~ **1275 POINTS**

* Because of the variability of assignments from week to week, point values associated with each module will not be the same, but range from 25-75 points per week.

APPENDIX A (continued)

Academic Dishonesty: This course will follow policies and procedures as outlined in the "Student Ethics and Conduct Code" section in the Student Handbook. Each and every student is responsible for his/her learning and is expected to follow individual or group work guidelines set forth for each activity and assessment in this course. If a student is found to have compromised his/her academic integrity, he/she will be referred to the Office of Student Services for disciplinary action.

Attendance Policy: IT IS MANDATORY THAT STUDENTS ATTEND ALL SCHEDULED SESSIONS in order to achieve their potential in the various skills. The faculty realizes, however, that certain extenuating circumstances may occur which would prevent attendance. This policy addresses those circumstances, the procedures for making-up work and allocation of points. Please read through this material carefully and direct any questions to the course directors. *It is the student's responsibility to comply with these policies, i.e.; course directors will not "track you down" to find out why you were absent.*

Switching Sections: SWITCHING SECTIONS IS NOT PERMITTED without prior consent of course directors, and is only allowed under extenuating circumstances.

Unexcused absence: Each unexcused absence will result in the **loss of 100 points** for that class session. It will be the responsibility of the student to make up any assignments for missed sessions. Students must follow the procedure for notification and make-up. Failure to arrange for make-up work within a time frame designated by the course directors and/or failure to make up the missed assignments will result in an *Incomplete Failure (IF)* for the course.

Excused Absence: Excused absences, anticipated and unanticipated, are based upon extenuating circumstances beyond the control of the student. Four areas fall into the category of extenuating circumstance: 1) medical necessity; 2) death of a family member; 3) pre-approved professional activities or 4) extenuating circumstances unforeseen by this policy.

1) Medical Necessity refers to unpredictable or serious illness of the student and his/her immediate family. Documentation, such as a medical statement from the patient's physician, may be required at the request of the course directors. Routine office visits within the control of the student are not considered extenuating and should be scheduled around the student's class.

2) Death of a family member refers to death of spouse, children or significant others within the immediate family including parents, grandparents and siblings of the student and/or spouse.

3) Pre-approved professional activities constitute an extenuating circumstance when the student and/or student organization has followed the appropriate notification procedures outlined in the School of Pharmacy Bulletin. It is the sole responsibility of the student to inform a course director of his/her planned absence **at least one month in advance**, preferably at the start of the semester. Documentation of attendance at the professional activity is required.

4) Extenuating circumstances: A course director should be contacted if a circumstance does not fall into one of the above categories. The decision of the course directors is final.

Procedure for Notification and Make-up Work: It is the sole responsibility of the student to notify the course directors of his/her absence. Once the student has met with a course director to discuss the absence and procedures for make-up work, the student will email a summary of the discussion to both course directors to ensure the student's understanding. Failure to do this and/or follow the procedures below will result in an unexcused absence and specified point penalty.

Anticipated absences: The student must notify a course director of an anticipated absence as early as possible **prior to absence**. If circumstances prevent the student from providing proper notification, he/she must arrange for another individual to contact a course director. Messages must include the student's name, social security number, scheduled class time and group number if leaving a voice or email message (see course director contact information on first page).

Unanticipated absences: Contact a course director within two academic business days following your return to arrange make-up work. Written documentation of the plan and the completed make-up work must be provided in a timely manner to the course directors.

Exceptions to these procedures will be made only under extraordinary circumstances as deemed appropriate by the course directors and/or the Scholastic Advancement and Appeals Committee. Students may initiate an appeals process through the Scholastic Advancement and Appeals Committee (outlined in the Student Handbook) for any circumstances they feel are extenuating and are not covered by this policy.

Tardiness policy: It is essential that all students are physically and mentally prepared at the time class begins. If you know you may be late prior to the class session, contact a course director. Tardiness penalties will be levied as followed:

1-5 Minutes	- 5 points
6-10 minutes	- 25 points
11-15 minutes	-50 points
> 16 minutes	-200 points

Dress Code: Students and course directors will be expected to dress in a professional manner while participating in the Professional Skills Development Course. The course directors, instructors and students (peers) are responsible for maintaining compliance with the dress code policy. Students not wearing clothing deemed appropriate by the course directors or instructor will be *penalized 15 points* for the first time. A second offense of this policy will result in the student being asked to leave and change into appropriate attire. Students asked to leave will be required to comply with the make-up work policy. The following are the guidelines for appropriate dress and follow those applied to the pharmacy environment:

Male Students: Short white lab coat, (long sleeves required, non-UCHSC logos and badges are not permitted), dress slacks, a collared shirt and tie.

Female Students: Short white lab coat (long sleeves required, non-UCHSC logos and badges are not permitted) skirt, dress (no more than 4 inches above the knee) or dress slacks, and a blouse or sweater. Jean skirts or dress is permitted.

Inappropriate dress includes: baseball caps, tight-fitting leggings/stirrup pants, spandex, any kind or color of jeans, shorts, tee-shirts, any type of sweat pants or sweatshirts, short skirts or revealing blouses, halter tops, tank tops, midriffs, back-less tops or fatigues.

APPENDIX A (continued)

STATEMENT OF UNDERSTANDING

I have thoroughly read the course syllabus for PHRD 3100. Upon completion of this reading I clearly understand and therefore have no questions concerning the course intent, content, policies, grading structure or dress code contained within this document. I understand that this document is an agreement between the course directors and each student and both parties agree to abide by the statements held within this document.

If questions arise as the course progresses, I clearly understand that it is my responsibility to ask the course directors for clarification.

Print Name_____

Sign Name_____

I have thoroughly read the course syllabus for PHRD 3100. Upon completion of this reading I have questions regarding one of the following items: the course intent, content, policies, grading structure or dress code contained within this document.

I have listed my question below and request further clarification.

Print name_____

Sign Name_____

Promoting Civility
from a New Faculty Member Perspective

Donna West

INTRODUCTION

As a new faculty member, you are excited about teaching. You are eager to do a good job. You spend hours preparing for a course. You begin to familiarize yourself with your new surroundings (lecture halls, faculty interactions, etc.), and about the time that trepidation and insecurity are beginning to abate and your comfort level rises, it happens.

- As you instruct the students to do a one-minute paper on the Friday prior to the week of spring break, a student yells from the back of the class, "You have got to be kidding me. This is SPRING BREAK. This is ridiculous."
- A student is sleeping in class. You direct a question to him and wake him. The student does not know the answer and is embarrassed. You emphatically remind him that he had better stay awake.
- You are lecturing when a student blurts out, "Are you single?" The class bursts into laughter.

Donna West, R.Ph., Ph.D., is Assistant Professor in the Department of Pharmacy Practice, College of Pharmacy Practice, University of Arkansas for Medical Sciences, 4301 West Markham, Slot 522, Little Rock, AR 72205 (E-mail: westdonnas@uams.edu).

[Haworth co-indexing entry note]: "Promoting Civility from a New Faculty Member Perspective." West, Donna. Co-published simultaneously in *Journal of Pharmacy Teaching* (Pharmaceutical Products Press, an imprint of The Haworth Press, Inc.) Vol. 9, No. 3, 2002, pp. 91-104; and: *Promoting Civility in Pharmacy Education* (ed: Bruce A. Berger) Pharmaceutical Products Press, an imprint of The Haworth Press, Inc., 2003, pp. 91-104. Single or multiple copies of this article are available for a fee from The Haworth Document Delivery Service [1-800-HAWORTH, 9:00 a.m. - 5:00 p.m. (EST). E-mail address: docdelivery@haworthpress.com].

© 2003 by The Haworth Press, Inc. All rights reserved.

- After class a student questions you about the relevance of the course to pharmacy and irritatingly states, "I had no idea that I had to sit through this crap to be a pharmacist."

The first incident happened to me in month three of the job, and the other three incidents were provided to me by other new teachers in colleges of pharmacy. Each one caught the faculty member by surprise. New academicians are usually not expecting these events to occur when they begin their teaching career. Unfortunately, it only takes a few incidents to decrease one's self-esteem or make one become indifferent to teaching (1).

New faculty members need to be aware of the potential for incivilities to occur, originating with both faculty members and students. Incivilities are words or actions that are disrespectful or rude (2). As illustrated above, they can be direct (e.g., verbal assault, inappropriate language) or indirect (e.g., sleeping in class, arriving late to class). The goal of this paper is to discuss methods and tools young faculty members can use to promote civility.

WHY ARE NEW FACULTY TARGETS FOR INCIVILITIES?

Incivilities seem to occur more often to new faculty members (3). It appears these incivilities can be attributed to both student and faculty causes. The students do not know the professor, and little is known about his or her reputation, grading, or exam format. Students often feel threatened by the unknown. Moreover, they want to test their limits and boundaries. When the new faculty member does not respond to these incivilities or responds inappropriately, the cycle of incivility begins.

Unfortunately, many new faculty members do little to promote civility. New faculty members often fail to establish rules and boundaries initially. For example, the new faculty member may fail to state, "No cell phones allowed in class. If you have one, put the ringer on vibrate and answer it after class." Then the cell phone rings in class and the student answers it, perhaps offending the new faculty member, but nothing is done. Some new faculty have unrealistic expectations (e.g., the student should respect me, pay attention to me) (4). When these expectations are not met, the faculty member, feeling threatened, attempts to remind the students who has the authority, resulting in incivilities. Furthermore, new faculty members want to prove themselves. They are eager and ambitious. Initially, an enormous amount of work may be given to students simply because the faculty member has so many ideas and wants to execute them all. Students may experience frustration and stress as a result, leading to uncivil behavior. It has been observed that some new faculty members do not assess students' prior knowledge of the subject, and, therefore, their lectures are too elementary or too advanced for the audience (3). Again, students become inattentive, bored, and frustrated. This usually leads to some form of acting out.

As stated by Dr. Berger earlier in this special edition, some professors experience incivilities more or less than others. This is true of new faculty members as well. Boice observed that regardless of faculty experience, immediacy and motivator valence seem to be major predictors of civility (3). Immediacy refers to the extent to which the professor gives verbal and nonverbal signs of warmth, friendliness, and general liking. Motivator valence refers to the use of positive (e.g., do you understand, you can do better) or negative motivators (e.g., what kind of question is that, obviously you didn't read). Professors who use positive motivators and have high levels of immediacy have fewer incivilities in their classrooms, as shown in Table 1. Successful senior teachers have learned to use positive motivators and have developed skills for expressing immediacy, while new faculty members are just beginning to develop these skills (3). New faculty members may unintentionally utter negative comments, give off condescending vibes, or become defensive, thereby fostering incivilities.

Whether incivility in education has worsened over the years is an interesting debate; however, understanding how to promote civility is more important. Young faculty members need to be aware of their own attitudes and behaviors. Moreover, they need to be prepared to foster civility as well as handle incivilities when they occur.

TABLE 1. Relationship Between Use of Positive Motivators and Level of Immediacy with Incivilities.

	% of motivators used positively by professor	Mean level of immediacy on 10-point scale
Young faculty who experience low incivility	81	6.2
Young faculty who experience high incivility	56	3.7

Adapted from Table 2 from Boice B. Classroom incivilities. *Res Higher Educ.* 1996; 37:453-586.

CHARACTERISTICS ASSOCIATED WITH CIVILITY

As Boice concluded, professors have a great deal of influence on whether incivilities occur in their courses (3). Although new faculty members cannot change students' behavior and are not responsible for students' behavior, they can exhibit certain characteristics that seem to diminish the possibility of incivilities occurring in the classroom. Immediacy and the use of positive motivators seem to overcome the lack of teaching experience.

As defined above, immediacy refers to the professor's ability to exhibit signs of warmth and friendliness. Behaviors associated with high and low immediacy are listed in Table 2 (3, 5). The signs of high immediacy indicate that the professor is approachable and cares. The professor respects the students as people who have needs and concerns. For example, starting and stopping class on time indicates respect for the students' time schedule. New faculty members should practice exhibiting signs of high immediacy. Coming to class early and asking students how they are doing or stopping to chat with a group of students in the hall indicates that one cares. When a student is meeting with a faculty member in his office, the faculty member should forward all phone calls and avoid other interruptions to indicate to the student that he or she is important. Additionally, new faculty should identify those behaviors associated with low immediacy that they exhibit and then try to change. For example, if a new professor tends to talk too fast, he could put reminders to pause or stop and ask for questions in his lecture notes.

Not only is it important to be friendly, but it is also important to motivate and encourage students. When faculty members are positive, inci-

TABLE 2. Examples of Behaviors Associated with Immediacy.

High Immediacy	Low Immediacy
• Displays eye contact • Moves around, looks for understanding • Smiles • Says hello to students outside of class • Leans forward • Listens to questions and concerns • Starts and stops class on time • Comes to class a few minutes early and stays a few minutes late to chat with students	• Talks too fast • No office hours–not available • Not attentive in office • Cancels class unexpectedly • Gives surprise quizzes or exam questions

vilities seem to decline. Encourage students by involving them in lecture, encouraging questions, providing positive comments and feedback, and being available outside of class. New faculty members have used blank index cards on the first day of class for students to indicate their pharmacy work experience, their hometown, and one concept they want to learn in the class. Other faculty members have used short surveys to learn about the students' preferences, interests, and experiences. These techniques enable faculty to involve the students and convey to them interest in their learning.

New faculty members should be aware of their own attitudes and behaviors, especially during the first couple of weeks (3). The first few weeks of the course are crucial, as the first impression is usually the one remembered.

PROMOTING CIVILITY

When preparing for a teaching position, there are four factors to consider in creating an atmosphere that promotes civility. These factors are likely to facilitate the development of immediacy skills and the use of positive motivators. The four factors are: find a mentor, prepare for classes, communicate your expectations, and get to know the students.

Find a Mentor

One of the most important recommendations is to find a successful teacher to serve as a mentor at the university where you are employed. This mentor can assist you in learning about the students at your university. Students at different institutions have different expectations, norms, and customs. For example, during the first week of class, a new instructor passed out the syllabus that included the semester project. She had already assigned students to groups. Students immediately began complaining. After class, she sought one of her colleagues to ask about group work and discovered that the students usually select their own groups because so many students commute and work. It is difficult for some of them to meet outside of class unless it is in the community where they live. A mentor reviewing the syllabus prior to distribution may have prevented this occurrence.

As mentioned previously, students seem to test their limits and boundaries with new faculty. Having a mentor can help you gauge when you are too tolerant or intolerant. Students may challenge you on attendance, grading, test schedules, or in-class time to work on projects. Having an experienced faculty member to talk to will assist you in making these decisions more reasonably. A mentor is also important when reading student evaluations that may contain personal comments (e.g., "get a new hairstyle") and other incivilities. A mentor can remind you that even the best teachers cannot please everyone.

Prepare

As a new faculty member, it is important to prepare for each lecture. Students will be wondering if this new professor really knows anything. If one seems indifferent to teaching and is not putting in the time to prepare, students will reciprocate. They, too, will become indifferent and not prepare for class, leading to boredom and incivilities. Also, the lack of preparation by faculty will not be respected by students.

Learning about different teaching methodologies and techniques is valuable. It is critical that new faculty learn how to assess students' prior knowledge and how to get students involved. Research has shown that involved students learn more and are more civil (3, 6). Examples of how to improve student involvement include one-minute papers, case studies, quizzes, small group exercises, debates, and in-class discussions (5, 7). When using these techniques, it is critical that faculty let students know what to expect and the purpose of the activity so the students do not feel confused or threatened.

There are numerous resources (e.g., books, AACP seminars) available to help new faculty members prepare for teaching. New faculty should discuss the resources available at their institution with their department chair or mentor. For example, at the University of Arkansas for Medical Sciences, young faculty can attend Teaching Scholars, a program that describes teaching concepts, including writing objectives, incorporating technology into the classroom, and developing active-learning exercises.

Both peer and student evaluations can also be helpful (8). It is recommended that new faculty members have peer evaluations annually. An objective outside observer can help identify areas that need improvement. Perhaps one is sending an unintended message nonverbally, talking too fast, or ignoring incivilities in the classroom. Although student evaluations often have inappropriate comments or material, there are usually a couple of "pearls" in each batch. Try to find those "pearls of wisdom" and incorporate them. For example, students continually complained about one faculty member being unavailable. This faculty member was off campus most of the time due to her clinical obligations. She now holds study sessions before the exam and has observed a decrease in the number of complaints about her inaccessibility. She commented that only a few students come to the help session, but the perception that she cares and is willing to meet with them is now there. In other words, she has increased her level of immediacy with the students.

Communicate Your Expectations

Because new faculty members are considered "unknown" by the students (What are the tests like? How does she grade?), it is important to establish and communicate class expectations, both academic and behavioral. These expectations should be stated in the syllabus as well as reviewed thoroughly on the first day of class (9). The syllabus should include course objectives, a course outline, expected academic performance, and evaluation criteria. Reviewing these on the first day of class will increase the likelihood that the expectations have been understood by the students (8). A poorly written syllabus that lacks clarity can lead to student frustration and anger.

It has been shown that incivilities increase when students are frustrated or under stress, especially during exam times or near deadlines for projects and assignments. Providing students with information about the exam format, the material covered by the exam, and the assignment parameters will help ease tensions. Providing help sessions, giving practice tests, and reviewing a preliminary draft of the report/project may also reduce incivilities.

A civility clause or other behavioral expectations should also be stated on the syllabus (8). If attendance is expected in your class, this should be stated. Again, talking with a mentor who understands the "general rules" for the college will help you understand how your expectations fit into the overall environment. With more students having electronic devices (e.g., cell phones, pagers, personal digital assistants), expectations regarding their use in your class or rotation should be stated.

It is helpful to explain why the rules exist. For example, a professor who states, "Please be on time. Coming into class 15 minutes late and crawling over others is disruptive and frustrating to me and your peers who are trying to learn," is likely to be better received than the professor who states, "Don't be late or else." The first message conveys to the students that the professor cares and is not just creating rules to establish authority. Presenting rules just to have authority can backfire and be perceived as threatening.

When communicating with students, new academicians should also be attentive to the nonverbal messages sent. How is it said? What is the tone of voice? Students may perceive certain words or actions as uncivil if the instructor is not careful. One faculty member continually snapped his fingers in class to quiet the students. The students perceived this to be demeaning and an attempt to control them, and it resulted in the students' continual chatting and uncivil behavior.

Get to Know the Students

Communicating with students is likely to improve student-faculty relations. As in all relationships, the better the relationship, the less incivilities occur. As Berger alludes to in the introduction, students may feel powerless and resort to passive-aggressive behavior and incivilities. To negate these feelings of powerlessness, provide students a way to communicate with you. E-mail the class requesting feedback, meet with representatives from the class to learn about their concerns and needs, provide feedback to students so they know how they are doing in the class, or conduct a mid-term teaching evaluation. When appropriate and feasible, compromise with the students (e.g., reschedule class time, change test).

Successful experienced teachers recommend learning students' names and getting to know them. Listed below are four examples of how to get to know students.

- One new faculty member learned the names of his 75 students in the first 2 weeks of class. Several students commented on this. They perceived that he must care if he learned all of their names, thus making it more difficult for them to objectify him.
- Several new faculty have gotten involved with student organizations (e.g., ASP, NCPA) and met the student leaders. The student leaders were able to provide a glimpse of what the class was thinking.
- One new faculty member included students by collaborating with them. She would ask students to collaborate with her on research projects. Other faculty encourage students to enter essay contests (e.g., NACDS Community Pharmacy Essay Contest) or other programs that involve both student and faculty participation.

- Some professors begin class with a famous quotation or a trivia question. These types of activities increase the interaction with students before lecture begins.

HOW TO RESPOND TO INCIVILITIES

Although new faculty can exhibit characteristics that seem to decrease incivilities, incivilities may still occur. Responding to them appropriately is the key to preventing or reducing future incivilities. As previously stated, the first few weeks are critical. Thus, responding assertively to incivilities is essential. Suggestions on how to handle incivilities are discussed in this section.

When incivilities occur, it is essential that the professor not blow up in anger but remain calm (5). Although it may be tempting, it is important not to return incivilities with incivilities. Instead, remain civil and be assertive.

In the first example provided (the student yelled that the assignment was ridiculous), the faculty member, using the broken-record technique, assertively restated to take out a sheet of paper for the one-minute paper. Most of the students were embarrassed, and when the faculty member controlled the situation calmly, the rest of the class did not contribute any other outbursts. Usually the majority of the class will disapprove of a peer's uncivil behavior, assuming the faculty member remains civil. When the students returned from spring break, the faculty member asked the student to come to her office. She expressed her disapproval of the behavior and set the rule that outbursts like that would not be allowed. If it happened again, a noncognitive (see Appendix A) would be written. The student apologized and stated he was only joking. There were no more inappropriate outbursts during the remainder of the course. The faculty member remained assertive in class but did not become angry or argue with the student. At the same time, she did not ignore the incivility. She addressed it with the person who performed the behavior. She reset the expectation. Ignoring it or laughing it off may have allowed for other types of outbursts to occur, whether jokingly or not.

Likewise, in the fourth example, the professor remained calm and assertively explained the relevance of the course. The professor was careful not to become defensive and engage this student in an argument. Instead, the professor listened to the student's concerns and then later tried to explain the importance and relevance of the material to the student.

Successful teachers not only treat incivility with respect but they also use it to their advantage (3). For example, a teacher may observe indirect incivility during class (e.g., shuffling papers, sighing, loud whispering) and sense the students' frustration. The teacher can use this as a sign to stop and review the material.

Faculty members are advised not to embarrass students publicly. Embarrassing one student may be perceived by the entire class as rude (9). If the class believes the faculty member has not been civil, the class dynamics will change: students will chitchat more, participate in class less, and become indifferent to the course (8). In the second example, the new professor made the mistake of embarrassing the student, which haunted him on his student evaluations at the end of the semester. Instead, the professor should have indirectly addressed the problem or responded to it politely (9, 10). It is usually best to see the individual after class to address the problem directly. In class, you can use humor or politely draw attention to the misbehavior (7). Examples of indirect ways to handle incivilities include leaving the front row open for late comers, walking near the person chit-chatting, or making direct eye contact. All of these actions send the message to the student that you are aware of his or her misbehavior.

Set clear boundaries and keep them (5). A physician stated that she clearly sets the boundaries when interacting with drug representatives. Every drug representative knows his or her ethical boundaries with the physician. Likewise, it is the faculty with authority in the student-faculty relationship, and it is their responsibility to set the boundaries. In the third example above, where the student asked the professor about her marital status, the faculty member immediately informed the student that this was an inappropriate question. After class, she reiterated to the student that his behavior was unacceptable. She also informed the department chair of the situation and sought advice.

When sexist comments are made or inappropriate behavior occurs, the faculty member must be assertive and state that this is inappropriate. For example, if a student makes a sexist comment, the faculty member may state, "I have been offended and feel disrespected. These comments and/or behaviors are not acceptable." Although it is tempting to ignore the incident and remain silent, this reaction will be interpreted as assent. Additionally, nervous giggling or laughing in response to inappropriate behavior will be interpreted as acceptance of the behavior. Then it is likely that the behavior or comments will occur again. Faculty members must speak out against inappropriate comments or behavior before the situation gets out of control.

Young faculty members must be careful not to give into pressure. Students may invite you to attend a party or grab a beer with them. Being a friend out on a Thursday night and being a teacher back in class on Friday is extremely difficult, if not impossible. It is suggested that faculty attend only the activities that are school sanctioned and be responsible. Be judicious in deciding what to attend and how long to stay. Even when attending school-sponsored activities, one should be attentive to the surroundings. One student began dancing in a provocative manner around a new faculty member at the annual college of pharmacy party. The faculty member quickly stated to the student to stop and walked away. The faculty member left the party to avoid any misconceptions.

It is important to remember that perceptions are reality. If other professors and students perceive you to be flirting with students or befriending students, it will be difficult to negate these perceptions or rumors. Often new faculty members lose the respect of many students when they attempt to become friends with some of the students and try "too hard" to be liked. Trying too hard to be liked in the classroom does not work either. Dropping the lowest grade or making the test easy to "make students happy" is only a very short-term solution to decreasing incivilities. In the end, most students do not respect this behavior.

Getting too involved with students can be professional suicide. In faculty-student relationships, mentor students and keep the boundaries clear. Students will appreciate and respect a faculty member who guides them and keeps the relationship unambiguous.

PERSISTENT INCIVILITY

It is advised that new faculty obtain a copy of the institution's policies and procedures (11). New faculty should become familiar with the rules, specifically those pertaining to incivilities. Appendix A provides an example of an incivility policy. This policy provides an effective mechanism for faculty to handle inappropriate behavior not related to academic performance. It should be noted that this policy not only deals with responding to incivilities but also provides a mechanism for faculty to reward students for good behavior.

Faculty members are advised to ask a mentor about the policies and procedures and the chain of command. Does the administration usually support the faculty? As a new faculty member, one wants to know that he or she is supported and that he or she is not guilty until proven innocent. After learning what the policies and procedures are, use them appropriately.

When problems persist, it is best to seek help, preferably from the department chair. Help with handling incivilities should be sought immediately, similar to the way the faculty member handled the "are you single" question and then sought the advice of the department chair in case the situation worsened. Department chairs, academic deans, and mentors can all provide guidance on how to deal with the situation (11). Following the chain of command and the institution's policies is important.

Each new professor must act on what he said he would do. For example, if the professor states that a noncognitive will be written up the next time it occurs, then a noncognitive must be written up if the incivility occurs again. It is also appropriate to warn a student that if the incivility occurs again, he or she will be dismissed from class. If the behavior occurs, then the student must be dismissed politely from class. Not dismissing the student only sends the message that you will tolerate the incivility.

CONCLUSION

It is evident that new faculty members who exhibit high levels of immediacy and use positive motivators can foster civility. New academicians should be friendly, treat students with respect, and communicate with students both in and out of the classroom. They should also encourage students and involve them in lectures using active-learning techniques. Stating the course expectations, both academic and behavioral, during the first lecture is also advised.

When incivilities do occur, new faculty members must not retaliate with incivilities. Instead, they should be assertive and communicate to the student(s) that the behavior is unacceptable. Likewise, when sexually derogatory remarks or other inappropriate remarks are made, the faculty member must not remain silent, but address the issue. Understanding the institution's policies and procedures with regard to incivility and seeking help from mentors and department chairs can be helpful when dealing with incivilities.

New faculty members should strive to promote civility in the classroom, remembering that experience is the best teacher. In fact, it is believed that developing a complex skill such as teaching requires approximately ten years of regular, deliberate practice before true expertise is achieved (12). When incivilities do occur, it is important to reflect, learn from the mistakes, and improve. The methods presented in this article can be used to prepare for and respond to incivilities appropriately.

Of utmost importance is the awareness of one's own behaviors and attitudes and the willingness to change those that promote incivility. Furthermore, it has been observed that faculty with an appreciation of incivility are least likely to experience it. In conclusion, the first step to promoting civility is to heighten awareness.

REFERENCES

1. Boice R. New faculty involvement for women and minorities. *Res Higher Educ.* 1993; 34:291-341.

2. Teaching Resources Center, College of Arts and Sciences, Indiana University, 2001. Available at http://www.indiana.edu/~teaching. Accessed 2001 Dec 18.

3. Boice B. Classroom incivilities. *Res Higher Educ.* 1996; 37:453-586.

4. Kuhlenschmidt SL. Promoting internal civility: Understanding our beliefs about teaching and students. *N Directions Teach Learn.* 1999; 77:13-22.

5. Berger BA. Incivility. *Am J Pharm Educ.* 2000; 64:445-50.

6. Johnson R, Butts D. The relationship among college science student achievement, engaged time, and personal characteristics. *J Res Sci Teach.* 1983; 20:357-66.

7. Newble D, Cannon R. A handbook for medical teachers. 3rd ed. Boston: Kluwer Academic Publishers; 1994.

8. Morrissette PJ. Reducing incivility in the university/college classroom. *Int Electron J Leadership Learn.* 2001; 5(4). Available at http://www.ucalgary.ca/~iejll/volume5/morrissette.html. Accessed 2001 Nov 28.

9. McGlynn AP. Incivility in the college classroom: Its causes and cures. *Hispanic Outlook.* 1999; (Sept 9):26-9.

10. Schneider A. Insubordination and intimidation signals the end of decorum in many classrooms. *Chron Higher Educ.* 1998; (Mar 27):A1-A14. Available at http://chronicle.com/colloquy/98/rude/background.htm. Accessed 2001 Nov 15.

11. Richardson SM. Civility, leadership, and the classroom. *N Directions Teach Learn.* 1999; 77:13-22.

12. Ericsson KA, Charness N. Expert performance: Its structure and acquisition. *Am Psychol.* 1994; 49:725-47.

RECOMMENDED READING

Boice R. Advice for new faculty members: Nihil nimus. Boston: Allyn and Bacon; 1999.

APPENDIX A

Scholastic Non-Cognitive Performance Evaluation
at the University of Arkansas for Medical Sciences-College of Pharmacy
(As Listed in 2001-2002 Student Handbook)

Scholastic non-cognitive performance is evaluated on the basis of certain demonstrated characteristics that are important to individuals preparing for a career in pharmacy. Characteristics included in these evaluations are attentiveness, demeanor, maturity, cooperation, inquisitiveness, responsibility, and respect of authority. Students shall receive a grade of "Outstanding" or "Inadequate" when appropriate. The lack of either grade indicates that the student has been judged to possess the demonstrated characteristics or that contact with the student has been insufficient to allow evaluation. Faculty members of each course in which the student is enrolled will make evaluations.

If the student receives two (2) or more grades of "Outstanding," the Associate Dean for Academic Affairs will notify the student in writing of the fact and will place a letter of commendation in the student's file.

If the student receives the grade of "Inadequate" in two (2) or more separate situations or incidents, the Associate Dean for Academic Affairs will undertake the following action (in the case of a serious violation, a single grade of Inadequate will suffice): (1) notify the student in writing that he/she has received an excessive number of "Inadequate" evaluations, (2) require the student to arrange a formal interview within one week with the individual(s) submitting the written report(s), and (3) will forward to the Scholastic Standing Committee the results of the interview, including the student's explanation for his/her behavior. The Scholastic Standing Committee may choose any or several of the following: (1) take no further action, (2) counsel the student in writing only, (3) interview and counsel the student, (4) interview and counsel the student and place him/her on leave of absence for an interval to be recommended by the Associate Dean for Academic Affairs and approved by the Scholastic Standing Committee, (5) interview and counsel the student and place him/her on scholastic non-cognitive probation for an interval to be recommended by the Associate Dean for Academic Affairs and approved by the Scholastic Standing Committee, (6) interview the student and recommend the student repeat the entire academic year, or (7) interview the student and recommend his/her dismissal from the College.

Dealing with Boundary Violations

Heidi M. Anderson-Harper

INTRODUCTION

This manuscript explores boundary violations and faculty groups who are particularly vulnerable to incivilities. Incivilities can occur between students and faculty because appropriate boundaries are not established between the two. As a result, when boundaries are violated, it becomes very difficult for faculty to use their expert power effectively and teach successfully. The first part of this chapter presents a framework explaining boundary violations as described by Peterson (1). Peterson describes the types of boundary violations that occur in a professional and client relationship, specifically violations of the relationship by the professional. These violations are presented in the first part of this chapter and related to the professor-student relationship. The second part of the manuscript describes violations that students make in the relationship (in and out of the classroom). The final section presents strategies faculty may use to establish boundaries to limit the likelihood of incivilities.

Boundary violations are the misuse of power in the professional-client relationship (1). Boundaries, as defined by Peterson, "are the limits that allow for a safe connection based on the client's needs. When these

Heidi M. Anderson-Harper, Ph.D., R.Ph., is Professor and Assistant Dean for Education Innovation, College of Pharmacy, University of Kentucky, 301B Rose Street, Pharmacy Building, Lexington, KY 40536-0082.

[Haworth co-indexing entry note]: "Dealing with Boundary Violations." Anderson-Harper, Heidi M. Co-published simultaneously in *Journal of Pharmacy Teaching* (Pharmaceutical Products Press, an imprint of The Haworth Press, Inc.) Vol. 9, No. 3, 2002, pp. 105-117; and: *Promoting Civility in Pharmacy Education* (ed: Bruce A. Berger) Pharmaceutical Products Press, an imprint of The Haworth Press, Inc., 2003, pp. 105-117. Single or multiple copies of this article are available for a fee from The Haworth Document Delivery Service [1-800-HAWORTH, 9:00 a.m. - 5:00 p.m. (EST). E-mail address: docdelivery@haworthpress.com].

http://www.haworthpress.com/store/product.asp?sku=J060
© 2003 by The Haworth Press, Inc. All rights reserved.
10.1300/J060v09n03_08

limits are altered, what is allowed in the relationship becomes ambiguous. Such ambiguity is often experienced as an intrusion into the sphere of safety. The pain from a violation is frequently delayed, and the violation itself may not be recognized or felt until harmful consequences emerge" (1). Simply stated, boundary violations invade the relationship between a professional and a client and exploit or destroy the trust that has developed. It involves a process–not just a single event–that grows like a cancer in the relationship and is not acknowledged until the dilemma has become serious (1). Peterson explains that "while violations fall on a continuum from minor mistakes to major transgressions, they all share the same characteristics. Learning to recognize the similarities gives us a map for deciphering potentially risky situations" (1).

Boundaries exist in the professional-client relationship to protect the relationship. It is the professional's responsibility to clearly identify and set these limits, as well as to maintain the limits so that the clients' needs are addressed above all else. When one extrapolates this to a teacher-learner situation, it suggests that teachers need to clearly define the boundaries for students and to recognize that if boundary violations arise, the relationship becomes unclear and may set the stage for incivilities. If a professor places his or her needs above those of the student, a boundary violation may occur, and the result may or may not be a civil situation. For example, the professor who takes credit for the work completed by one of her students violates the trust that has developed. This lays the foundation for erosion of the relationship.

CHARACTERISTICS OF BOUNDARY VIOLATIONS

This section describes Peterson's characteristics of boundary violations and gives examples of incivilities resulting from professor-student violations. All examples presented are based on actual situations involving women and minority professors. However, the situations are disguised to protect the identity of the individuals and the school.

The four characteristics of boundary violations are: (1) *a reversal of roles*, (2) *a secret*, (3) *a double bind*, and (4) *an indulgence of professional privilege*. These characteristics are interrelated in a system that has its own existence. Let's look at each of these characteristics in more detail. First, when the professional and client switch places or the professional places his or her needs above the clients', *a role reversal* has taken place. For instance, when a professor schedules office hours for students and then repeatedly shows up late or not at all, the professor places the student's needs in a secondary role. Although, this may appear as a minor violation, the professional (teacher) is still responsible for defining the parameters of the relationship and determining whose needs will come first and who will meet them. In another serious situation, the professor befriends the students in a cordial manner and joins them for several "nights on the town." Later, the students perform poorly on an exam given by the same professor and expect some special consideration from the professor. They are shocked when the professor takes a professional role and does not treat them in the friendly way they had come to expect. Clearly, roles have been confused and the students find the circumstances ambiguous. The professor has created a situation in which the students do not receive consistently fair treatment. A definite boundary violation, role reversal, has occurred.

The second characteristic, *the secret*, involves hiding information that is harmful to the client, thus destroying the trust that has been built in the relationship. "In a boundary violation, the presence of secrets functions either (1) to separate the client from the professional while deceitfully maintaining the pretense of a common endeavor or (2) to falsely join the client and professional against those who are on the outside and do not know the secret" (1).

Peterson asserts, "More important than the content of the secret, though, is its effect on both the professional and the client. A secret splits rather than strengthens the bond of trust. It protects behaviors that are not legitimate to the intent and purpose of the professional-client relationship by restricting the client's access to knowing. Because the professional acts out of the secret rather than out of regard for the client's need, a part of the professional's self is not available to engage with the client." An example of the secret is when the professor dates a student who is in her class, then attempts to maintain a neutral position toward this student during classroom encounters. This puts the student in an ambiguous situation, thus giving rise to the boundary violation, the secret.

The third characteristic, *the double bind*, as described by Peterson places the client in a conflict of interest (1). It involves the professional placing his or her needs above the client's, thus causing the client to lose in the relationship because trust is violated. The client feels that he or she has no choices in handling the situation. The client feels "indebted to the professional for his or her help, they worry that they will betray the relationship if they comment on the violation. The guilt, along with the real fear of possible abandonment by the professional, blocks them from taking action. On the other hand, their continuing participation in a violation risks their integrity, because they fail to give credence to their inner voice that says something is wrong" (1). Thus, the client feels used and feels that he or she has compromised his or her own needs. The result is a loss of respect for oneself.

Peterson further expounds, "Boundary violations place clients in untenable binds. Since they are highly dependent on the professional, clients feel both trapped inside the relationship and bound by their perceived inability to move independently. They are tied both by what they need from the professional and by their fear of being without the relationship. If they give up the relationship, they lose the professional's needed expertise. If they stay in the relationship, they lose a part of their personhood" (1).

In one situation, a professor attempted to use his close relationship with one student (Student A) to gather information about another student (Student B). Student A was taking an elective course with the professor because she had an interest in this area as a career endeavor. This professor was well known for his expertise in the area, and she was honored that he had agreed to help her develop her interest and possible career focus. After working with him for a complete semester, Student A developed a close relationship with the professor. In another course, this professor had given various writing assignments to the class. The professor noticed that one student in particular appeared to have submitted a paper that he probably had not written (based on previous papers that this student had written). He noticed that Student A had a close relationship with Student B. Because of his relationship with Student A, he asked her to ascertain whether Student B had actually written the paper or had received it from the Internet or another source. Of course, the professor requested that Student A do this in a concealed fashion and report the information back to him so that he had evidence to change the grade. Although Student A felt she was compromising her integrity and loyalty, she also felt compelled to honor this request because she was taking the special elective, needed a good grade, and was depending on the professor's expertise to help her achieve her career goals. In this case the boundary violation involves both the secret and the double bind.

The final characteristic, *the indulgence of personal privilege*, involves the professional taking advantage of the personal information that he or she has obtained from the client during their encounters. Peterson describes this characteristic:

In every boundary violation, there is a fit between the professional's need and the client's vulnerability. This coupling produces the opportunity for the professional to take advantage of the client. Indeed, since the professional has the authority over and the responsibility for the client's situation, he or she is particularly susceptible to extending the privilege of his or her superior position and intruding on the client. The professional's decision to act on this opportunity grows out of his or her presumption that he or she can use his or her privilege to do whatever he or she wants with the client. Once the professional substitutes his or her agenda for the ethos of care, his or her energy is directed toward an illegitimate goal. He or she operates out of a different place internally . . . The indulgence of personal privilege allows the professional to pursue the relationship for his or her own purposes. (1)

In situations where the professional violates this indulgence of personal privilege, he or she often uses language such as, "It is in the best interest of the client that . . ." or this is being "done for the client" (1). The violator rationalizes inappropriate behavior and violation of the professional-client relationship. Further,

Since the purpose of the professional-client relationship is to serve the client, however, professionals who extend their privilege have to establish a legitimate claim to intrude and some reason to explain behavior that is otherwise incongruent with the ethos of care. They have to persuade themselves that their behavior is either inconsequential or helpful and necessary for the client. In effect, they must hide their true impulses. (1)

As these examples illustrate, every boundary violation damages the professional-client relationship. It is imperative, therefore, that professionals keep this in mind and not allow violations to betray the trust that has formed between them and their clients.

STUDENT VIOLATIONS OF BOUNDARIES

Students also violate boundaries in the professor-student relationship. These violations may lead to minor or major incivilities. This section presents examples of real-life situations where students have violated boundaries. Suggestions for handling these situations are offered.

The Grade or Exam Challenger

Some students use their own poor performance to attack professors by arguing that the teaching was inadequate or the grading was unfair, thus contributing to their poor performance on the exam. In my early years as a professor, I allowed students to challenge grades on exams. Often these challenges were almost belligerent. When I returned the exams, I explained my detailed grading policy and the item analysis of each question (even the open-ended questions), but I still had these less-than-respectful challenges. I would become quite defensive. Finally, I developed a grade challenge policy, which was also detailed in my course syllabus. This policy required students to write a challenge letter within 24 hours after an exam was returned if they wished to dispute a grade. Whenever they challenged an exam, they had to write a letter indicating why they believed that their answer was graded inappropriately, they had to provide evidence in the letter that clearly justified their response, and they were not to disturb the teaching assistants or me about the matter because they would receive a written response from me. After implementing this policy, I not only received fewer complaints, but the level of civility regarding exams changed. Students became more civil and I became less defensive through the setting of boundaries.

The Flatterer or Con Man (or Woman)

Some students like to "sweet talk" professors by giving them compliments such as "you're the best professor I ever had"; "you always dress so nice and better than other professors"; or "I am impressed with the depth of your expertise." For some faculty, these compliments overshadow their ability to sense that the student is really seeking to enhance his or her grades, get deadline extensions on assignments, or receive favoritism. Faculty must tread carefully and be cautious in these situations while remembering to consider possible hidden agendas.

The Overtly Hostile Student

Some students are known for attacking the professor's point of view publicly in class. It is not the disagreement that is the problem, but the lack of respect. Others violate boundaries by becoming confrontational, disrespectful, or angry. In these cases, a faculty member would be wise to listen carefully, to acknowledge the student's feelings, to state the faculty member's position clearly and rationally, and to avoid becoming defensive. If necessary, meet with the student in the presence of another (possibly senior) faculty member outside of class.

The Expertise Challenger

You may come across those students who will challenge the expertise of the professor, a guest, or other lecturer. Unfortunately, the literature states that students challenge the expertise of women faculty more often than male faculty. A situation cited to me involved a female course coordinator who arranged various speakers in her class on a variety of subjects. She asked the class to evaluate each presenter at the end of the presentations. During one particular class, she invited a male presenter and a female presenter to the same session. During this session, the male presenter was unprepared, was unorganized, and had difficulty relating the material to the objectives in the course. However, the students stated that they enjoyed his humor and unrelated stories. On the other hand, the female presenter was more professional, was better organized, used stories that related to the material, and summarized the main issues throughout the session. Upon reviewing the evaluations, it was evident to the professor that there was a major difference between the student's evaluations of the male presenter versus the female presenter. The male presenter received a reasonably high to moderate evaluation in this situation; however, unless the female lecturer "did a song and dance and had incredible content and a great personality," she was more likely to receive critical remarks on her evaluation no matter how well prepared or qualified she was. In fact, students were more likely to treat female presenters in a more uncivil manner than male presenters.

As these situations imply, when faculty fail to provide clear boundaries, it is apparent that problems may arise. Such problems can lead to incivilities and, if they persist, to frustration on the part of students and faculty.

According to Richardson, student incivility in higher education is appearing more often in news reports and popular literature (2). What are the implications for faculty? Who are the most vulnerable faculty? What can faculty do to prevent incivilities? Faculty who receive uncivil student behavior can become stressed, discontented, and burned out. Faculty who have previously faced uncivil actions may begin devoting time and energy to planning coping strategies and not focus on content and class material. The faculty member may go to class and become defensive even before any inappropriate behavior occurs. In fact, some faculty become so frustrated that they may dread going to class altogether and become demoralized and disillusioned with teaching.

Appleby asserts that uncivil behavior on the part of faculty or students can also jeopardize the learning process for those students not involved in the irritating or inappropriate behavior (3). Inappropriate behaviors can create a stressed environment for the other students, and learning becomes counterproductive when incivilities obstruct learning opportunities (4).

Morrissette argues that:

> Faculty members who are trained in the helping professions may be more prepared to discuss problems that emerge in the classroom due to their experience and familiarity with unexpected client behavior. For example, it is not unusual for helping professionals to experience client resistance, confrontation, or anger within a counseling context. Therefore, faculty with clinical experience who encounter similar behavior in the classroom may be better equipped to employ their clinical skills in handling or diffusing troubling situations. (4)

Although clinical faculty may be used to dealing with client behavior, new clinical faculty are inexperienced as teachers and may not be comfortable handling these types of situations within the classroom.

Several years ago, a pharmacy faculty member shared a situation with me in which a student did not believe in the new pharmaceutical care philosophy of practicing pharmacy. This student verbally and nonverbally discarded the professor's strategies and activities in the class by citing his own experiences in the community pharmacy in which he had worked. The student further conveyed hostility toward the professor, challenged her authority publicly in the classroom, and made it clear that the new faculty member was not only younger but also obviously had not been practicing in the "real world." Unfortunately, the faculty member became so overwhelmed that she failed to set boundaries in the class and lost control for the entire semester. Students started skipping class or were loud and failed to treat her with respect when they were in class. She later became so disillusioned with teaching that she returned to practice. There are several strategies she should have tried before leaving teaching. For example, she could have discussed the situation with a senior faculty member to get ideas for handling the students. Of course, she should have met with this particular student outside of class. Further, she should have set clear expectations about how she wanted students to behave during her class. Finally, she could have invited practicing professionals into the class to validate the concepts she was teaching.

Which faculty are the most vulnerable? Royce responded in her keynote presentation at a campus forum on academic incivility that the most vulnerable are "[y]oung faculty, women, faculty of color, faculty who do not reside in the 'most favored nation' departments, faculty who invest time in community- rather than individual-building activities. Those faculty need to be supported because we would be the poorer without their voices and their talents. That support has to be consistent, tangible, vocal and visible" (5).

Lieberg stresses that there are differences with women faculty in the classroom (6). "For instance, women faculty members are expected, by students, to act more supportive and motherly than male professors, but if they do, students are less likely to see them as strong and intellectual teachers. If women hold to tough standards, they are viewed as being 'masculine.' Women are more likely to be challenged" (6).

Cannon describes her experience as a new female faculty member:

> When I started, I was reluctant to address the emotionally laden content of the classroom. But over time, I gave more and more attention to classroom interaction, which, like all group interactions, is structured by inequalities of power among the participants. They are not random, haphazard, or out of the control of the teacher. Our behavior as faculty members and the way we structure our courses play major roles in the nature of classroom interactions as they unfold throughout the semester. (7)

FACULTY AND ADMINISTRATION RESPONSE TO INCIVILITIES

How Can Faculty Respond?

What can faculty do to prevent incivilities? Faculty can reduce the chance of incivilities in the classroom by setting boundaries and making students aware of these boundaries. As Cannon suggests, faculty must recognize that the interactions in the class are not random or out of the professor's control. Faculty must set the limits and boundaries. Consider the following strategies.

Set Limits and Explain Rules Clearly. Set boundaries by spelling out the rules for your class in the course syllabus. For example, you might explain the type of courtesy behavior you expect when a guest is visiting the class or lecturing. Describe the consequences of inappropriate behavior such as talking during lectures, arriving late to class, or reading the newspaper during class. Spend time in the very first class period reviewing the syllabus with special attention to these rules and limits. The advantage of a well-written syllabus is to clearly communicate your expectations to students.

Address Problem Behavior Directly and Immediately. Often when problems occur it is easy to ignore them. Although ignoring the problem may avoid class distractions or public confrontation, it does not eliminate the problem. Unresolved conflicts can resurface and cause major problems later.

Model Appropriate Behavior. If you want students to be prompt, courteous, respectful, organized, etc., model these behaviors. Don't arrive to class late. Don't keep students over the allotted class time and then expect them to act appropriately. Don't yell, embarrass, or use public humiliation if you want students to be courteous and respectful. Don't present material and assignments in a disorderly fashion and expect students to be organized.

Get Mid-Term Feedback. Ask students to give input about the course during the mid-term. This allows you to correct problems, to respond to students' needs, and to defuse potential incivilities. One approach developed by Redmond and Clark at the University of Washington in 1982 involves using small focus groups of students to provide feedback at mid-term (8). Students respond to three questions during the focus group discussion:

- What elements in this course helped you to meet the learning objectives?
- What elements in this course prevented you from meeting the learning objectives?
- What specific suggestions do you have to improve the course?

How Can Administrators Respond?

Administrators have various ways to respond to incivilities, including being supportive; offering advice; listening; and, when necessary, providing strategies to reduce the chance of incivilities occurring. Department heads need to provide the necessary support and resources to allow faculty to be effective teachers in the classroom. When incivilities occur, the department chair should take time to discuss the matter with the faculty member, listen to both sides of the situation, and offer suggestions as appropriate. The key role for the department head is to reduce the stress and awkwardness that the faculty member feels in these situations.

To prevent incivilities from occurring, department chairs should take a more proactive approach with new and inexperienced faculty. The majority of new faculty have not had any formal preparation on how to be college teachers. Several strategies may help these inexperienced faculty members:

- Assign a senior effective teacher to serve as a teaching mentor to the new faculty member. This individual can offer help with a variety of issues and concerns.
- Assist the faculty member in developing clear expectations and policies for the course.
- Provide peer observation and/or peer reviews for the individual to gain insights from another faculty member. Observations should only be done by invitation.
- Talk with faculty about their behavior in the classroom and their ability to set a good example.
- Offer suggestions to those faculty who indirectly promote uncivil behavior by their own behavior. For instance, some faculty can provoke an unpleasant situation by publicly humiliating or invalidating students or by making snide remarks, and some faculty can be arrogant and blinded to their contribution in the situation.

Lastly, to prevent student-faculty conflicts from escalating, department heads should have a grievance process in place and make sure that students and faculty are familiar with the process.

As a last resource, deans need to be prepared to step in when the situation warrants upper-level action. For example, one minority faculty member described her experience in a predominately nonminority student classroom. When she entered class on several occasions and approached the overhead projector to place her materials for the day, she would come across upsetting racial material or comments that had been written on the projector. Other students told her that several students in the class were leaving these notes, but they refused to identify the individuals. After she reported these incidents to the department head and expressed her feelings about the situation, the department head simply minimized the situation and indicated that she needed to toughen up. In another situation, the minority female faculty received upsetting racial telephone calls at her home from students. Of course, she was both frightened and uncomfortable. In this case, the dean called a meeting of the entire student body and publicly informed the students that such behavior would not be tolerated in that school.

Administrators must provide the support and resources to allow faculty to be effective teachers. This may involve assisting faculty with uncivil situations and providing guidance to avoid potential problems. It is also important that administrators realize these are very sensitive circumstances. Finally, administrators need to respond quickly and appropriately to make sure that the faculty member feels like a valuable asset to the school.

CONCLUSION

Although incivilities in college classrooms are increasing, we must not lose heart. We must remain vigilant to the reason we became college professors. Parker Palmer expresses it well:

> Many of us became teachers for reasons of the heart, animated by a passion for some subject and for helping people learn . . . We lose heart, in part, because teaching is a daily exercise in vulnerability . . . As we try to connect ourselves and our subjects with our students, we make ourselves, as well as our subjects vulnerable to indifference, judgment, ridicule. To reduce our vulnerability, we disconnect from students, from subjects, and even from ourselves. We build a wall between inner truth and outer performance and we playact the teacher's part. Our words, spoken at remove from our hearts, become the "balloon speech in cartoons" and we become caricatures of ourselves. We distance ourselves from students and subject to minimize the danger–forgetting that distance makes life more dangerous still by isolating the self. (9)

REFERENCES

1. Peterson Marilyn. At personal risk: Boundary violations in professional-client relationships. New York: W. W. Norton & Company; 1992.

2. Richardson S. Promoting civility: A teaching challenge. *N Directions Teach Learn.* 1999; 77:i-vi.

3. Appleby D. Faculty and student perceptions of irritating behaviors in the college classroom. *J Staff Program Organ Dev.* 1990; 8:41-6.

4. Morrissette PJ. Reducing incivility in the university/college classroom. *Int Electron J Leadership Learn.* 2001; 5(4). Available at http://www.ucalgary.ca/~iejll/volume5/morrissette.html.

5. Royce AP. Civility: An uncommon good. Keynote presentation at Campus Forum on Academic Incivility, Indiana University, Bloomington, IN, October, 1998. Available at: http://campuslife.indiana.edu/Civility/program/keynote.html.

6. Lieberg C. Help for bad manners in the classroom. *TALK.* 1996/1997; 1(4). (Newsletter published by the Center for Teaching, University of Iowa). Available at: http://www.uiowa.edu/~centeach/talk/volume1/bad-manners.html.

7. Cannon LW. Fostering positive race, class, and gender dynamics in the classroom. In: Teaching and learning in the college classroom. Feldman KA, Paulsen MB, eds. ASHE Reader Series. Needham Heights, MA: Ginn Press; 1994:301-6.

8. Redmond M, Clark D. Small group instructional diagnosis: A practical approach to improving teaching. *AAHE Bull.* 1982; 34(6):8-10.

9. Palmer P. The courage to teach. San Francisco: Jossey-Bass; 1998.

Index

http://www.haworthpress.com/store/product.asp?sku=J060
© 2003 by The Haworth Press, Inc. All rights reserved.

SPECIAL 25%-OFF DISCOUNT!

Order a copy of this book with this form or online at:
http://www.haworthpress.com/store/product.asp?sku=4914
Use Sale Code BOF25 in the online bookshop to receive 25% off!

Promoting Civility in Pharmacy Education

___ in softbound at $14.96 (regularly $19.95) (ISBN: 0-7890-2121-8)
___ in hardbound at $26.21 (regularly $34.95) (ISBN: 0-7890-2120-X)

COST OF BOOKS _____

Outside USA/ Canada/
Mexico: Add 20% _____

POSTAGE & HANDLING _____
(US: $4.00 for first book & $1.50
for each additional book)
Outside US: $5.00 for first book
& $2.00 for each additional book)

SUBTOTAL _____

in Canada: add 7% GST _____

STATE TAX _____
(NY, OH, & MIN residents please
add appropriate local sales tax

FINAL TOTAL _____
(if paying in Canadian funds, convert
using the current exchange rate,
UNESCO coupons welcome)

❑ **BILL ME LATER:** ($5 service charge will be added)
(Bill-me option is good on US/Canada/
Mexico orders only; not good to jobbers,
wholesalers, or subscription agencies.)

❑ **Signature** _____

❑ **Payment Enclosed: $** _____

❑ **PLEASE CHARGE TO MY CREDIT CARD:**

❑ Visa ❑ MasterCard ❑ AmEx ❑ Discover
❑ Diner's Club ❑ Eurocard ❑ JCB

Account #_____

Exp Date _____

Signature_____
*(Prices in US dollars and subject to
change without notice.)*

PLEASE PRINT ALL INFORMATION OR ATTACH YOUR BUSINESS CARD

Name	
Address	
City	State/Province	Zip/Postal Code
Country	
Tel	Fax
E-Mail	

May we use your e-mail address for confirmations and other types of information? ❑Yes ❑No
We appreciate receiving your e-mail address. Haworth would like to e-mail special discount
offers to you, as a preferred customer. **We will never share, rent, or exchange your e-mail
address.** We regard such actions as an invasion of your privacy.

Order From Your Local Bookstore or Directly From
The Haworth Press, Inc.
10 Alice Street, Binghamton, New York 13904-1580 • USA
Call Our toll-free number (1-800-429-6784) / Outside US/Canada: (607) 722-5857
Fax: 1-800-895-0582 / Outside US/Canada: (607) 771-0012
E-Mail your order to us: Orders@haworthpress.com

Please Photocopy this form for your personal use.
www.HaworthPress.com

BOF03